Principles of Medical Professionalism

Principles of Medical Professionalism

Gia Merlo
New York University, NY, USA

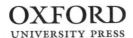

OXFORD
UNIVERSITY PRESS

OXFORD
UNIVERSITY PRESS

Oxford University Press is a department of the University of Oxford. It furthers
the University's objective of excellence in research, scholarship, and education
by publishing worldwide. Oxford is a registered trade mark of Oxford University
Press in the UK and certain other countries.

Published in the United States of America by Oxford University Press
198 Madison Avenue, New York, NY 10016, United States of America.

CIP data is on file at the Library of Congress
ISBN 978-0-19-750622-6

DOI: 10.1093/med/9780197506226.001.0001

1 3 5 7 9 8 6 4 2

Printed by Marquis, Canada

Contents

Preface

As a practicing psychiatrist for over 25 years, I have treated many physicians and their families. I first began developing the concepts of this book in the 1990s when I was in private practice in Philadelphia after transitioning from academia at the University of Pennsylvania. Helping physicians and their children for decades helped me to consolidate my view that, while most physicians inherently want to help patients and society, many have very limited understanding of the ramifications of their choosing to enter medical school. Why is that? What can they do about it? How does this gap affect patient outcomes and their personal well-being?

Helping physicians who transgressed professional boundaries to adjust to the new normal and redevelop their professional identities, and helping their families deal with the potential humiliation of public and professional reprimand, was often challenging. The pain and suffering was real and often so unnecessary. Many of these physicians had gone down the "slippery slope," unaware of the violations they were committing that later evolved into serious transgressions. I studied these issues as a clinician for many years and was pained for my patients and all those who were impacted. The children, the patients, and the spouses all suffered. Sometimes I treated those far removed from the initial problem, and other times, children of substance-abusing physicians, those who underwent sexual violations, and physician's spouses who gave up on their marriages because their spouse was suffering from moral distress, compassion fatigue, burnout, or undiagnosed depression.

There were multiple themes that I observed in the physicians that I treated. These included a loss of focus on happiness and self-care, struggles with professional and personal communication, difficulties understanding how to work in a team, and questions about their life's purpose and their faith. These existential questions are important to reflect on for all members of society, and working through them is a task required of ongoing personal and professional growth. However, due to the heavy time commitment of physician's training and work, these reflective tasks often never made it to the top of the to-do list. In addition, many of these physicians had learned to compartmentalize their suffering throughout their careers as a result of being socialized in the culture of perfection that has historically pervaded the medical profession. The professional taboo of "what happens when we make a mistake" was all too real. For physicians who often strived to excel in every endeavor, discussing and working to address personal transgressions was often difficult, if not impossible.

Most physicians start medical training with above average coping strategies and mental health compared to their peers in college. I was able to observe this first-hand as I taught the foundations of this book to premedical students at Rice University. The students helped me refine my understanding of the developmental underpinning of physicians' character traits and of their service orientation and intentions prior to entering medical school. I then started teaching medical professionalism in 2015 to a variety of audiences including medical students, residents, and practicing physicians. While teaching at Baylor College of Medicine, I continued to be impressed with the professionalism I observed across the board.

Why this book then? The literature overwhelmingly indicates that there are significant problems present in the medical profession. One problem is the physician burnout epidemic, which is cited to affect one in two physicians. While these issues have many causes, and are largely systemic, what is apparent to me is that it would serve us well to better educate our physician workforce to develop a more resilient professional culture. However, I, and other medical educators, have found that medical professionalism can be difficult to teach explicitly. With this thought in mind, I wrote this book, *Principles of Medical Professionalism*, which is intended to serve as a guide to help physicians develop a professional identity that incorporates happiness and self-care: a professional identity that is inherently more resilient to the challenges in our profession.

Many of the topics presented in the book have been discussed in the literature, but the framing of these chapters is based on my clinical experience and teaching. Each chapter shares a common theme of happiness and self-care as a vital component of medical professionalism. While the organizational structure of this book may not seem intuitive at first blush, it is designed to give readers opportunities for informed reflection. For example, artificial intelligence is likely to dramatically change our roles as physicians in the future, a concept I discuss early on in the book. These changes are likely to affect many of the paradigms of medicine, but I believe that physicians will continue to add value to this equation through the physician–patient relationship by delivering the "soft skills" that are a vital part of medical professionalism. The importance of these soft skills—such as empathy, compassion, and communication—are discussed throughout the book, allowing readers the opportunity to reflect on what it means to be a medical professional while considering their changing roles as physicians.

Through my experiences in child psychiatry and early practice of clinical psychiatry, I developed a sense that my work as an educator is to impart foundational knowledge, model self-reflection, share my lived experiences, and embrace my humanness to facilitate growth and depth in thinking of the learners. In his theory of cognitive development, Piaget suggests that our learning is limited by our cognitive abilities, which follow stages but are nevertheless fluid. This principle has shaped my teaching methodology. For example, in my classroom, I often use dramatic patient stories to teach about medical professionalism and then share my gut reactions and verbally reflect on the material. These stories serve to inspire my students to re-evaluate their biases and cognitive lacunae and embrace the cognitive dissonance that is created. This "space" of psychological disequilibrium allows for growth— learning, questions, relearning, and rebalancing with a different equilibrium. This is the same pedagogical model I follow in the book. By presenting information that many physicians and medical learners may not be familiar with, and providing opportunities for reflection, I hope that the reader can integrate this information into their professional identity.

After reading this book, I hope that health professionals of all levels will feel empowered with practical knowledge, tools, and techniques that will allow them to become more competent caregivers and leaders in their field. Indeed, the ultimate goal of the book is to encourage a medical educational framework supporting personal and professional transformation that may lead to more resilient and happier physicians. Thus, physicians may be better equipped to attend to the tasks of patient care that incorporates attention to healing, caring, and compassion while upholding their duty to serve the patient and society.

Acknowledgments

This book is the outcome of a process that has involved many people. First and foremost, I am grateful to my patients over the years who have trusted me to partner in their care. I am humbled and grateful for the lessons being a physician continues to afford me.

I am deeply indebted to Dick and Sylvia Cruess for their mentorship and many conversations that solidified my thinking around medical professionalism. The selfless commitment of time and focus by John Coverdale and Toi Blakely Harris was so appreciated, especially John's endless Sunday 7 AM meetings at my dining table (thank you, Mary Coverdale!). I have also benefited tremendously from the input I received from many colleagues in Houston at Rice University and Baylor College of Medicine including Jennifer Blumenthal-Barby, Timothy Boone, Audrea Burns, Trevor Burt, Dan Carson, Cindy Farach-Carson, Arnaud Chevallier, Elizabeth Festa, the late Malcolm Gillis, Jane Grande-Allen, Joseph Kass, Jim Lomax, Nancy Moreno, Colleen Morimoto, Alana Newell, Kristen Ostherr, Adam Pena, Peter Rossky, Paula Sanders, Daryl Shorter, Geeta Singhal, and Moshe Vardi. I am also thankful for the physicians at Houston Methodist Hospital, who exemplify medical professionalism.

I would also like to thank my colleagues who are devoted to medical professionalism education including Julie Agris, Marco Antonio de Caralho Filho, Joseph Carrese, Jennifer Chevinsky, David Doukas, Neil J Farber, Ellen Friedman, Liz Gaufberg, Patricia Gerber, Michael Green, Fred Hafferty, Valerie Harris Weber, Tom Harter, Macey Henderson, Patrick Herron, Andrea Leep Hunderfund, Craig Klugman, Barbara Lewis, Janet Malik Weinstein, Maggie Moon, Dennis Novack, Raul Perez, Leann Poston, Saleem Razack, Preston Reynolds, Steve Rosenzweig, John Spandorfer, Carol Stanford, Rebecca Volpe, and Laura Weiss Roberts. Several physicians in the Philadelphia community, at the University of Pennsylvania, and UT Southwestern in Dallas were important in my early professional development including Salman Akhtar, Tami Benton, Ira Brenner, Jennifer and Jay Bonovitz, Rhoda Frankel, Carmen Harlan, Urszula Kelley, Paul Mohl, Kathie

Trello-Rishel, Annie Steinberg, David Steinman, Jutta Vogt, and the late Elizabeth Weller.

Additionally, I would like to thank my New York University colleagues including Lisa Altshuler, Sean Clarke, Emerson Ea, Helen Egger, Kim Glassman, Trace Jordan, Adina Kalet, Perri Klass, Beth Latimer, Fidelindo Lim, Penelope Lusk, Charlie Marmar, Linda Mills, Carol Morrow, Alan Schlechter, Jess Shatkin, Eileen Sullivan-Marx, and David Stern for providing a stimulating academic community.

I have taught medical professionalism to students at Rice University, the Baylor College of Medicine, and New York University. All these cohorts of students have given me a wealth of their insightful perspectives into the subject matter of this book over the years and I am tremendously grateful to each and every one of them. This journey has helped me solidify my own understanding of what this book should be about and how it should be framed. Over the years, I am especially grateful for the contributions from Elizabeth Festa, Paul Ryu, and Griffin Milan. I am also grateful to my teaching and research assistants in my Medical Professionalism class at Rice including Hannah Abrams, Andrea Amaro, John Michael Austin, Rohan Bhardwaj, Deeksha Bidare, Cylaina Bird, Monica Bodd, Claire Bonnyman, Tristan Boss, Taylor Brooks, Stephanie Cho, Wesley Chou, Cierra Duckworth, Ola Elechi, Margeaux Epner, Jovany Franco, Sofia Gonzalez de Corcuera, Abby Gordon, Ruchi Gupta, Hannah Hanania, Jing He, Marisa Hudson, Trevor Jamison, Saiesh Kalva, Amritha Kanakamedala, Rohit Kavukuntla, Erin Kilbride, Erin Kim, Amy Kuprasertkul, Caroline Lee, Komal Luthra, Griffin Milan, Ranjini Nagaraj, Ariyaneh Nikbin, Olivia Nixon-Hemelt, Maya Pai, Rohan Palanki, Claire Peng, Ethan Perez, Tri Pham, Kathryn Pickrell, Karen Qi, Emily Rao, Simran Rahman, Saisree Ravi, Jacqueline Rios, Paul Ryu, Dhanatcha Sadetaporn, Charles Sauve, Jessica Sheu, Siyu Shi, Shweta Sridhar, Anagha Srirangam, Arlen Suarez, Christine Tang, Julie Thamby, Hannah Todd, Serena Tohme, Puja Tripuraneni, Marjada Tucker, Jessica Weng, Aliza Wolfe, Cathy Wu, Erik Wu, Victoria Yuan, Caroline Zhu, and Nadia Zulfa.

Thank you to the editorial team at OUP and especially to Andrea Knobloch for believing in the project early on and trusting my capacity to deliver. Finally, I owe a huge debt of gratitude to my husband, Antonio Merlo. Were it not for his persistence and steady encouragement, this book would have never seen the light of day. And to my sweet, loving, passionate daughter Monisha Lewis, I am tickled by the miracle of your life and awed by the power of your hands. Thank you.

1

A Roadmap to Medical Professionalism

To become a medical professional is to have navigated a specified course of advanced education, prepared academically, and emerged with a longing to accept a career path in the pursuit of a higher purpose for the good of society and themselves.[1]

Medical professionalism encompasses the proficiency, skills, competence, and effectiveness with which professionals conduct themselves in the practice of their chosen profession. Medicine is a challenging career, but the medical professional can not only survive, but excel throughout the years-long process of intense studying, late nights and early mornings, moments of uncertainty in life-or-death situations, "difficult" patients who may refuse or forget about their recommended treatment, and on-call nights where everything seems to go wrong. Indeed, it is challenging to be a physician. However, for most physicians, the satisfaction and joy associated with serving patients far outweigh the challenges that they face. Those who have demonstrated their ability as critical thinkers, appreciate the principles behind medical professionalism, and show self-awareness and the ability to grow from their failures and successes have a greater capacity to reap the benefits associated with being a physician.

Becoming a member of the medical profession is not a matter of passing milestones but of embodying the values, behaviors, and identity of a physician. Forming a professional identity requires, however, that you hone your skills as an observer and, even more significant, as an engaged, reflective person. Understanding and internalizing professionalism and reflecting on your role in the profession are not simple tasks. This book, read thoughtfully and with an open mind, will help you on your journey toward being a conscientious, professional physician.

Challenges of and to professionalism

Medical professionalism is challenging to define. If you search for a definition, you are sure to find a long list of impressive personal qualities, behaviors, and competencies that capture an inspirational—almost superhuman—ideal. Some definitions, such as those advanced in the Physician Charter of the Medical Professionalism Project,[2] present a detailed list of values, traits, and behaviors. These include adherence to high ethical and moral standards and demonstration of a continuing commitment to excellence. Others succinctly summarize the many discrete manifestations of professionalism by calling for "the habitual and judicious use of communication, knowledge, technical skills, clinical reasoning, emotions, values, and reflection ... for the benefit of the individual and community being served."[3p226]

All of these various definitions recognize that professionalism is "more than a demonstration of isolated competencies."[3p227] Thinking holistically about professionalism not only changes how we understand its individual dimensions, but also acknowledges that professionalism is necessarily greater than the sum of these parts. One cannot overestimate the importance of this quality amidst the inherent uncertainty of so many situations that physicians must negotiate. Unquestionably, medical professionals have an obligation to look after their patients. The physician–patient bond is a fiduciary relationship in which patients must place their faith in the abilities and intentions of their physicians, and, in return, physicians must act in their patients' best interests *even at a cost to themselves*. Yet, this exchange is often easier said than done.

You may encounter values and behaviors that conflict with the definition of professionalism and work against your own best efforts to maintain it. These discrepancies are known as the *informal* and the *hidden* curricula, and they can have a significant impact on your development:

- The *informal curriculum* covers exchanges of information and uncensored commentary of faculty, staff, and other colleagues that take place outside of the classroom, lab, or other formal academic settings, such as in the elevator, corridors, the lounge, cafeteria, or the on-call room. For instance, you may witness role models violating a patient's confidentiality, making derisive comments about a patient's race or ethnicity, making fun of a patient, or critiquing other colleagues.

- The *hidden curriculum* encompasses organizational policies, decisions, and customary practices that reveal a different political and values system at work than the one that is formally acknowledged. You may note that certain tenets of professionalism are valued over others, for example, prioritizing time spent completing paperwork over time spent with patients.[4] In some cases, professionalism may be interpreted as loyalty to the academic hierarchy as opposed to a promise to society. In such a scenario, "covering up minor mistakes is far more likely to be evaluated as 'professional' than will other avowed professional values such as honesty and respect for patients."[4p1011]

Institutions may inadvertently reveal the value they place on professionalism in their handling of (or failure to handle) lapses in it. When institutions have systems in place to effectively work through infractions, complaints are more likely to be lodged, and difficult situations dealt with to the satisfaction of all involved. When few, or none, of these systems are in place, the message is clear: you report at the peril of yourself and your colleagues, so it might be best to remain silent. However, silence causes small offenses to fall by the wayside, often causing serial offenders to become so entrenched in their wrongdoing that—by the time the administration is forced to act—there is no way to remediate their behavior adequately.

The hidden curriculum also pervades institutional identity in less obvious ways. The choices that medical schools make in selecting their curriculum, shaping their promotional materials, establishing evaluation methods, allocating their budget, and discussing their programming also suggest their priorities.[5p15] These decisions do not necessarily indicate nefarious motivations, but show an institutional opacity that contrasts with the transparent ideals of professionalism as currently defined.

Challenges to professionalism are certainly not limited to the training arena. It's not surprising that part of the current focus on physician professionalism in the educational environment came about, in part, because of increased public scrutiny of the profession. Medical professionalism hasn't necessarily deteriorated since the mid-20th century, but media of all kinds have brought infractions to the public's attention. Although the cases that have gained the most media attention are far from representative, their sensational status has elevated their importance. In one, a man who discovered that his phone had accidentally recorded his colonoscopy found that his operating team had insulted him while he was unconscious and that his anesthesiologist had described his diagnosis as "a shot in the dark."[6] Clearly, incidents of this type are devastating for a society's trust in the benevolence and empathy of its physicians. Medicine's regulating bodies take swift action to prevent similar incidents from occurring and restore confidence in the profession, but often once it has happened, harm cannot be rectified.

Structural aspects of today's healthcare system are also prone to scrutiny. Media reports of healthcare costs and negative outcome rates have led the medical community to undertake further self-examination. If action is not rapid enough (or where even physicians cannot effect much change, such as in matters of insurance or hospital pricing), other players become involved. Outside of the realm of state and federal governments, regulating committees such as the American Medical Association and state medical licensing boards are allowed to decide on the proper code of conduct for physicians as well as which physicians are qualified to practice. When the public becomes displeased with the performance of the medical profession, the government often is called on to act to protect the common good. Although they may have good intentions, legislators and executives rarely have any experience in providing healthcare, patient care, insurance claims, or undergoing the process of maintenance of certification and continuing medical education.

As one example, administrators and policymakers are more involved in healthcare decision-making than ever before. These decision makers are often distanced from the impact and repercussions of their decisions, as many of us have observed during the COVID-19 pandemic. For example, decisions on how to ration personal protective equipment, allocation of hospital bed space to sick patients, and uncertainty around hospital policies regarding physicians who become ill are often made at a corporate level with limited physician input. At the same time, clinicians responded with exemplary medical professionalism even during a time of great uncertainty. Physicians often need to weigh the pros and cons of focusing on self-care versus their obligation to society, a concept that we discuss in more detail in Chapter 3 of this volume. Further thoughts on the physician's role as an employee will be provided in Chapter 16 of this volume.

For better or for worse, medicine has been continuing to move in the direction of the separation of the roles of clinician and financial decision maker. It is important to understand that there will always be political, economic, and managerial factors that influence the provision of care. To do best by their patients and themselves, medical professionals must make sure their voices rise as decisions get made about the future of healthcare. This kind of engagement is equally important in maintaining physicians' powers of self-governance: one of the essential tenets of professionalism. For quality improvement measures and medical processes to continue to be in the hands of those with the most experience, physicians must fastidiously maintain exemplary professionalism.

The commitment to maintain professionalism, amid a variety of pressures and challenges, has made its way down the medical hierarchy and into medical schools. There is an ongoing effort to devise better methods for imparting the fundamental tenets of medicine to future physicians, as well as a continuing struggle to determine when students have achieved mastery. Recent studies suggest that lapses in student professionalism in medical school correlate with future infractions associated with disciplinary action. For instance, one study led by Papadakis and colleagues shows that "twice as high a proportion of disciplined physicians as of control physicians demonstrated unprofessional behavior in medical school."[7p2676] What can medical schools do to better prepare graduates and help prevent future disciplinary actions from occurring? One option is to incorporate professionalism into the curriculum and work with students who have lapsed to remediate and hopefully improve their behavior. Many medical schools are beginning to utilize both of these strategies.

Another option that is gaining traction with medical schools to improve the professionalism of their graduates is to strike at the root of the problem: the medical school application process. They have tried to select for moral maturity and other traits that indicate a predisposition for professional behavior.[8] While grade point average and Medical College Admission Test scores are strong indicators of a student's potential for success in medical school, admission officers have long recognized that these two numbers don't tell the entire story. Personal statements and interviews can give medical schools an idea of an applicant's ability to reflect on past events and demonstrate an understanding of issues affecting the profession and society as a whole, as well as his or her proficiency in communication and introspection.

Although these characteristics are by themselves crucial components of professionalism, some admissions offices have sought to standardize this process through a different method: the multiple mini-interview (MMI).[9]

The MMI requires applicants to complete several short interactions at separate stations, each of which is assessed by a different reviewer. Some of these interactions are similar to those an applicant might confront in a traditional interview, such as questions about their motivation to pursue medicine or about ethical issues (e.g., "Should placebos be given to patients?"). Others may test an applicant's critical thinking under pressure (e.g., "Is it reasonable to believe aspartame causes multiple sclerosis?") or ability to engage with a hypothetical situation (e.g., a coworker refuses to fly to a conference because of past trauma).[10] This flexible interviewing model allows reviewers to assess communication skills in a more practical way, such as through a scenario with an actor playing the role of a disgruntled patient or a small group project in which applicants must complete a task together.[8] One of the more significant advantages of the MMI is that it enables reviewers to measure an applicant's spontaneity and ability to adapt to unexpected scenarios in a high-stress environment. As such, the MMI aims to approximate the pressures that applicants may encounter in medical school and later in the profession.

Professional identity formation

While the movement toward MMI offers one promising approach to gauge an individual applicant's critical thinking ability and interpersonal skills, it does not address the myriad of topics covered in a comprehensive professionalization program. This book assumes that all students can benefit from a curriculum that builds on their self-awareness and socialization as these develop during their undergraduate years, forging connections between the curriculum and experiential learning, the individual, and the broader community. This process is called professional identity formation (PIF).[11]

Professionalization, as a process of identity formation, has not always been the norm in the field of medical education. In a recent article that portrays current pedagogical controversies and the curriculum and assessment of the frameworks focusing on medical professionalism, Irby and Hamstra discuss PIF as a framework in relationship to two earlier professionalization frameworks: the virtue-based approach and the behavior-based approach.[12] The virtue-based sense of professionalism emphasizes the personal qualities, beliefs, and character traits of exemplary physicians. "Internal habits of the heart"[11p1607] not only testify to the moral and ethical compass of the individual physician but also inform current professional guidelines, such as those that govern ethical confidentiality and clinical best practices such as effective doctor–patient communication.

Not surprisingly, as Irby and Hamstra note,[12] virtue is quite challenging to assess. For this reason, medical educators developed a second model that identifies measurable proxies for these values. This behavior-based model identifies discrete, carefully delineated, and progressive sets of behaviors that manifest a student's growth into a competent, ethical, and caring physician. In other words, the model seeks to identify what a physician does as a measure of what he or she believes, thinks, and feels. We can easily see the influence of these models in current definitions of professionalism. The behavior-based model is still the dominant framework in medical education.[11p1607]

However, the behavior-based model is imperfect, because it runs the risk of minimizing the complexity and nuance of professionalism by reducing it to a checklist of traits and standard operating procedures. Medical professionalism necessarily transcends such lists and uniform characteristics.[12] Instead, it ought to be "the motivational force—the belief system—that leads clinicians to come together, in groups and often occupational divides, to create and keep shared promises."[13p713] A sense of accountability and self-regulation at the level of the community is crucial to maintaining trust, especially as new policies, regulations, and technologies reshape the healthcare field.

This need for a broader belief system that can reinforce accountability and self-regulation has prompted recent interest in PIF. Professional identity can be interpreted as a "representation of self, achieved in stages over time during which the characteristics, values, and norms of the medical profession are internalized,"[11p1447] and its formation, in medical school and beyond, is paramount to a physician's professionalism amidst challenging circumstances. To be clear, PIF does not eschew teaching and assessing values and behaviors; instead, it makes these values and behaviors more relevant by embedding them in a framework that "socialize[s] learners into thinking, feeling, and acting like a physician" through "participation in a community of practice."[12p1608] If we developed a shorthand description of the three frameworks, we might think of the virtue-based context as one that emphasizes *knowing*; the behavior-based, *doing*; and PIF, *being*.[11p1448]

In its mission of promoting a state of being, PIF draws upon many of the same pedagogical methods that shaped earlier curriculum strategies, including facilitated discussions, case studies in ethics, reflective writing, and role modeling.[12p1609] PIF departs from earlier methods in foregrounding positive role modeling as a means of affecting socialization. Group work, dialogue, feedback, and coaching play are also instrumental in fostering a spirit of communal growth. Students themselves must be active participants in this process, and the PIF framework presumes an "aspirational" stance concerning professional identity.[12p1609] In this vein, PIF offers a refreshing departure from predominantly achievement-based assessment approaches. While these types of assessments are certainly here to stay, they do little to indicate progress in developing professional identity. PIF is not a matter of memorization and regurgitation: it requires receptivity, a spirit of anticipation, and an openness to change.

The theory of PIF acknowledges that internalizing a belief system does not occur overnight, but is, in fact, a lifelong process. Our understanding of this process has been shaped by the influential work of Cruess, Cruess, and Steinert, [14] who themselves drew from work by Piaget and Inhelder, Kohlberg, Erikson, Kegan, Marcia, and others in the field of developmental psychology. Erikson states that, generally, identity formation is the primary psychological process that happens during adolescence.[15] According to this model, people construct their identity in adolescence as they deal with a crisis between identity and role confusion. Marcia expands this model by defining four different statuses in which adolescents occupy according to their progress in the process of identity formation: identity diffusion, identity foreclosure, identity moratorium, and identity achievement.[16]

The concept of identity formation within the medical profession draws heavily upon the theories of Robert Kegan. He described the evolution of professional identity in terms of movement across a set of stages, some of which an individual might never reach.[17] At the early stage of the *instrumental mind*, individuals express a more limited view of their environment and exhibit a strong desire for external validation. As they progress, individuals attain a more *socialized status* in which they demonstrate an awareness of the expectations of the group to which they aspire to belong and attempt to meet these expectations. Developing still further, they may reach the *self-authoring mind* stage in which they can examine the values of their communities with a more critical eye and begin to form a sense of their unique persona within an organization. The final (and most elusive) stage, the *self-transforming mind*, describes those highly evolved individuals who draw upon and intersect a variety of frameworks for understanding the world while remaining aware of the limitations of these structures; they are further able to manage complex and contradictory information without disorientation.

Kalet and colleagues adapted Kegan's stages of development for use in a study of identity formation among first-year medical school students as illustrated in Table 1.1.[18]

The students were asked to complete a professional identity essay to measure their progression against Kegan's model of identity evolution. These questions addressed the medical profession and their place in the community, such as "What does being a member of the medical profession mean to you?" and "What would be the worst thing for you if you failed to live up to the expectations of your patients?" They further completed the Defining Issues Test that evaluated their inclinations in responding to moral problems.[18p256] They discovered that more than half of the students were at the instrumental or socialized stages, only a very small percentage had reached the self-authoring stage, and no students had attained self-transformational status.[18p258] This might seem disheartening at first glance, but it confirms students' malleability even at the graduate level and validates the project of addressing identity formation much earlier in a student's development. Students are likely be in the instrumental or socialized stages. This is not only understandable but also expected. According to Kegan's stages of professional development, perfection is not the goal, nor is it expected.

Another useful model to use when thinking about the process of PIF is Miller's pyramid. It was originally postulated in 1990 and recently amended by Cruess, Cruess, and Steinert as illustrated in Figure 1.1.[19]

In the medical profession, Miller's pyramid has had a lasting impact in shaping how we assess physicians and physicians in training. In its original formulation, there are four levels (Knows, Knows How, Shows How, and Does) through which medical professionals move as they develop their professional identity. At the lowest level, *Knows*, the physician is building the foundational knowledge base necessary to be a professional, which ranges from basic anatomy to epidemiology to ethics. At the *Knows How* level, the

Table 1.1 Kegan's Stages: The Four Broad Levels of Mental Complexity Relevant to Professional Medical Education

The Instrumental Mind[a] (Stage 2)	This stage is characterized by external definitions of self, a predominance of *either-or* thinking, limited perspective-taking ability, and an emphasis on the mastery of technical skills. This stage is characteristic of adolescence and early adulthood.
Transition (Stage 2/3)	This stage involves increase ability to have perspective, to learn organizational norms from others, and to emphasize mastery beyond technical skills.
The Socialized Mind (Stage 3)	This stage is characterized by increased social perspective-taking ability among allies or one's in-group members. Understanding and expectations of the professional role is externalized, shaped by interpersonal relationships, observing others, and following the norms and status quo within organizations without question. Some adolescents and most adults are in this stage.
Transition (Stage 3/4)	This stage is characterized by a greater understanding of one's self in the professional role and greater awareness of choices in dealing with influences that work against a professional's integrity.
The Self-authoring mind (Stage 4)	This stage involves the ability to *step back enough from the social environment to generate a seat of judgment or personal authority that evaluates and makes choices about external expectations.* The independence of judgment and problem-solving abilities of stage 4 translates to greater fidelity to one's sense of self within the professional role. At stage 4, one can discern negative social influences that can erode one's professional identity and integrity. Effectiveness within high-level professional or leadership roles requires stage 4 capacities.
Transition (Stage 4/5)	This stage one can understand and reconcile multiple contradictory ways of thinking and being.
The Self-Transforming Mind (Stage 5)	This stage is characterized by the ability to examine one's self-authored personal authority, recognize the limits of any one system of constructing meaning, and seek out novel or alternative systems. A recognition of the interdependencies of different system or ways of being and an ability to reconcile contradictory or seemingly paradoxical ways of constructing meaning is a hallmark of the emergence.

From A. Kalet, L. Buckvar-Keltz, V. Harnik, V. Monson, S. Hubbard, R. Crowe, H.S. Song, and S. Yingling, "Measuring Professional Identity Formation Early in Medical School, *Med Teach* 39, no. 3 (2017): 256, reprinted by permission of the publisher (Taylor & Francis Ltd. http://www.tandfonline.com).
[a]Stage 1 is qualified as childhood.

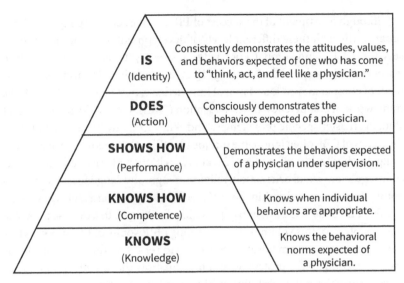

Figure 1.1 The amended Miller's pyramid that includes professional identity formation.

From R.L. Cruess, S.R. Cruess, and Y. Steinert, "Amending Miller's Pyramid to Include Professional Identity Formation," *Acad Med* 91, no. 2 (2016): 180–185. Copyright © 2016. © 2016 by the Association of American Medical Colleges.

physician takes that knowledge and develops an understanding of how to use it. For example, given a list of patient symptoms, the medical professional can make a diagnosis and suggest an appropriate treatment. At the *Shows How* level, physicians can put their understanding into action. At this point, they can integrate their knowledge and skills to deliver successful care in the clinic. You may think that this is the final goal, but in fact, the *Does* level is the ultimate objective wherein physicians function independently to deliver a high standard of care.

The 1990 Miller's pyramid measures medical *competency* as a set of standards to reach and master, but evolving definitions of medical professionalism include the concepts of a never-ending process of professional identity formation.[20] Cruess and colleagues suggested adding a new level to the apex of the 1990 Miller's pyramid, titled *Is*.[19p181] At the peak of the pyramid, physicians have internalized how to *think, act, and feel like a physician* and now organically display this newfound evolving identity. At the *Is* level, physicians not only exhibit the professionalism and clinical skills of the *Does* level but live it.

Although assessment of the success of PIF involves categorizing a student's progress through these different levels of development, it is not meant to assess the basic foundational knowledge necessary to ensure that medical learners can proceed to the next stage in their education. At this time, assessment of competency in foundational knowledge is best achieved through the framework of competency-based education (CBE). CBE seeks to ensure that students master specific proficiencies and skills. In many instances, however, the rigors of CBE often ignore the unique identities that medical professionals bring to the healthcare system. Diversity (whether of race, ethnicity, age, ability, gender, sexual orientation, religion, geography, language, or socioeconomic status) is valued within the profession, because it contributes to societal equality and adds to the mission of providing healthcare to a diverse populace (see Chapter 7 of this volume). The governing philosophy of PIF supports this mission in prompting medical professionals to reflect on the individual identities they bring to the profession and imagine how they meld with others as they advance through their training. This identity formation process is necessarily messy and requires students to venture into uncharted and, at times, uncomfortable terrain as they negotiate the parts of their identities that don't readily fit into this new framework. PIF is, nonetheless, a crucial part of the process of professionalization and serves to create a distinct range of experience from which the medical professional can draw for a lifetime.

The road ahead

In October 2017, the World Medical Association, an international confederation of more than 10 million physicians from 114 nations, unanimously voted to revise the Geneva Declaration, a modern successor to the Hippocratic Oath, to include the clause, "I will attend to my own health, well-being, and abilities in order to provide care of the highest standard." As the practice of medicine enters the modern era, a combination of disruptive factors, including the increased use of electronic health records and changes to the U.S. healthcare system, have left physicians struggling to find happiness in their careers. While systemic changes are necessary, doctors are beginning to realize that they have also neglected self-care, a crucial aspect of medical professionalism. This neglect may be contributing to alarming rates of physician burnout, depression, and suicide.

The reflective process and its life-long value is discussed in Chapter 2 of this volume. Each of the subsequent chapters frames the values of medical professionalism by describing a unique facet of the profession, and provides strategies for the reader to consider and reflect on their personal beliefs and explore their current and future role in the profession (see Chapter 16).

One of the main goals of the book is to inform future physicians and current practitioners that being a medical professional is not about being perfect, but rather about being human and recognizing their own limitations (see Chapter 3). Learners can manage their expectations about the profession while becoming more resilient to disruptions in the medical field such as artificial intelligence (see Chapter 4) and the changing patient–doctor relationship (see Chapter 5).

The Flexner Report, published in 1910, has often been noted to be instrumental in the transformation of medical education both positive and negative. It helped set admission and graduation standards to pass specific knowledge and attitudes surrounding medicine from physicians to students. However, currently, trainees are expected to rely on the example of professors and close mentors to develop their professional identity in what is referred to as the hidden curriculum. Although largely successful, this tradition has proven insufficient and, in many instances, unreliable, because the success of many medical students and residents still depends on their ability to "catch on" to informal aspects of training. Due to this educational gap and lack of support, students, residents, and physicians may encounter issues during medical practice, including boundary violations (see Chapter 5), declines in empathy (see Chapter 6), physician burnout (see Chapter 10), depression and suicide (see Chapter 11) and substance use disorder (see Chapter 12). It is also important to note that the Flexner Report, which caused the closing of all but two historically Black medical schools, in addition with other systemic forces, have arguably contributed to discriminatory practices in the field of medicine, leading to a need for cultural praxis and social justice (see Chapter 7).

Medical professionals must also understand the importance of team-based care (see Chapter 8); the impact of religion, spirituality, and humanism in healthcare (see Chapter 13); and the concerns that have arisen due to the aging physician workforce (see Chapter 15). Financial planning is another aspect of medical education that has long been neglected (see Chapter 14), as has been the value of preventative care and addressing chronic diseases through the evidence-based emerging field of lifestyle medicine (see Chapter 9).

This book is intended to serve as a guide for physicians as they develop their professional identity by encouraging them to reflect on who they are and who they want to become. In particular, the book's emphasis is on how and *why* physicians ought to focus on self-care, happiness, and well-being as they advance through the process of socialization into the medical community of practice.

Chapter Quick Summary

- Medical professionalism is more than demonstration of individual competencies; it includes embodying the values, behaviors, and identity of a physician through a process of professional identity formation.
- Observation and the reflective process are key skills in forming a professional identity.
- The challenges of professionalism in the current institutional organization renew demands on physicians to fastidiously maintain exemplary professionalism.
- Encountering values and behaviors that conflict with the definition of professionalism can work against physicians' best efforts. A discussion on the *informal* and *hidden* curricula and how they can have a significant impact on professional development can address this problem.
- All learners can benefit from a curriculum that scaffolds their self-awareness and socialization, forging connections between the curriculum and experiential learning, the individual, and the broader community.
- PIF broadens the scope of study for medical learners independent of the rigors of CBE strategies.
- This book is intended to serve as a guide for physicians as they develop their professional identity by encouraging them to reflect on who they are and who they want to become.
- This book focuses on the values of self-care and happiness and their importance for physicians.

Resources

Frost, H.D., and G. Regehr. "'I Am a Doctor': Negotiating the Discourses of Standardization and Diversity in Professional Identity Construction." *Acad Med* 88, *no.* 10 (2013): 1570–1577.

Hafferty, F. W. "Beyond Curriculum Reform: Confronting Medicine's Hidden Curriculum." *Acad Med* 73, no. 4 (1998): 403–407.

Jonsen, A.R., C.H. Braddock III, and K.A. Edwards. "Professionalism." *University of Washington School of Medicine*. 2014. https://depts.washington.edu/bhdept/ethics-medicine.

Papadakis, M.A., A. Teherani, M.A. Banach, T.R. Knettler, S. L. Rattner, D.T. Stern, J.J. Veloski, and C.S. Hodgson. Disciplinary action by medical boards and prior behavior in medical school. *New Engl J Med* 353, no. 25 (2005): 2673–2682.

"Patient Records Doctor's Insults during Surgery, Wins $500,000 Lawsuit." *ABC Eyewitness News*. June 24, 2015. http://abc13.com/health/listen-patient-records-doctors-mocking-him-during-surgery/802568/

References

1. Callaghan, J. "Professions and Professionalisation." In *Encyclopedia of Critical Psychology*. Edited by T. Teo, 1509–1515. New York: Springer, 2014.

2. Medical Professionalism Project. "Medical Professionalism in the New Millennium: A Physicians' Charter." *Lancet* 359, no. 9305 (2002): 520–522. https://doi.org/10.1016/S0140-6736(02)07684-5

3. Epstein, R.M., and E.M. Hundert. "Defining and Assessing Professional Competence." *Jama* 287, no. 2 (2002): 226–235.

4. Brainard, A.H., and H.C. Brislen. "Learning Professionalism: A View from the Trenches." *Acad Med*, 82, no. 11 (2007): 1010–1014.

5. Hafferty, F.W., and B. Castellani. "The Hidden Curriculum." In *Handbook of the Sociology of Medical Education*. Edited by Maureen T. Hallinan. New York: Springer, 2009.

6. Jackman, T. "Anesthesiologist Trashes Sedated Patient—And It Ends Up Costing Her." *Washington Post*, June 23, 2015. https://www.washingtonpost.com/local/anesthesiologist-trashes-sedated-patient-jury-orders-her-to-pay-500000/2015/06/23/cae05c00-18f3-11e5-ab92-c75ae6ab94b5_story.html

7. Papadakis, M.A., A. Teherani, M.A. Banach, T.R. Knettler, S.L. Rattner, D.T. Stern, J.J. Veloski, and C.S. Hodgson. "Disciplinary Action by Medical Boards and Prior Behavior in Medical School." *New Engl J Med* 353, no. 25 (2005): 2673–2682.

8. Bebeau, M.J., and V.E. Monson. "Guided by Theory, Grounded in Evidence: A Way Forward for Professional Ethics Education." In *Handbook of Moral and Character Education.* Edited by Larry Nicci, Darcia Narvaez, and Tobias Krettenauer, 557–582. New York: Routledge, 2014.

9. Eva, K.W., H.I. Reiter, J. Rosenfeld, K. Trinh, T.J. Wood, and G.R. Norman. "Association Between a Medical School Admission Process Using the Multiple Mini-interview and National Licensing Examination Scores." *JAMA* 308, no. 21 (2012): 2233–2240.

10. Eva, K.W., J. Rosenfeld, H.I. Reiter, and G.R. Norman. "An Admissions OSCE: The Multiple Mini-Interview." *Med Educ* 38, no. 3 (2004): 314–326.

11. Cruess, R.L., S.R. Cruess, J.D. Boudreau, L. Snell, and Y. Steinert. "Reframing Medical Education to Support Professional Identity Formation." *Acad Med* 89, no. 11 (2014): 1446–1451.

12. Irby, D.M., and S.J. Hamstra. "Parting the Clouds: Three Professionalism Frameworks in Medical Education." *Acad Med* 91, no. 12 (2016): 1606–1611.

13. Wynia, M.K., M.A. Papadakis, W.M. Sullivan, F.W. Hafferty. "More Than a List of Values and Desired Behaviors: A Foundational Understanding of Medical Professionalism." *Acad Med* 89, no. 5 (2014): 712–714.

14. Cruess, R.L., S.R. Cruess, and Y. Steinert. *Teaching Medical Professionalism: Supporting the Development of a Professional Identity.* 2nd ed. New York: Cambridge University Press, 2016.

15. Erikson, E.H. *Identity, Youth and Crisis.* New York: Norton, 1968.

16. Marcia, J. E. "The Empirical Study of Ego Identity." In *Identity and Development: An Interdisciplinary Approach.* Edited by H.A. Bosma, T.L.G. Graafsma, H.D. Grotevant, and D.J. de Levita, 67–80. New York: SAGE, 1994.

17. Kegan, R. *The Evolving Self.* Cambridge, MA: Harvard University Press, 1982.

18. Kalet, A., L. Buckvar-Keltz, V. Harnik, V. Monson, S. Hubbard, R. Crowe, H.S. Song, and S. Yingling. "Measuring Professional Identity Formation Early in Medical School, *Med Teach* 39, no. 3 (2017): 255–261.

19. Cruess, R.L., S.R. Cruess, and Y. Steinert. "Amending Miller's Pyramid to Include Professional Identity Formation." *Acad Med* 91, no. 2 (2016): 180–185.

20. Kumagai, A.K. "From Competencies to Human Interests: Ways of Knowing and Understanding in Medical Education." *Acad Med* 89, no. 7 (2014): 978–983, https://doi.org/10.1097/ACM.0000000000000234

2
The Reflective Process

The role of reflection in professional identity formation

In medicine, we often think of the term "reflection" within the scope of its dictionary definition, as "careful thought about something, sometimes over a long period of time." While this definition is useful, this chapter discusses reflection within a specific framework. Fundamentally, reflection is about thinking through past situations and gaining from retrospection and introspection. The medical professional can use reflection to enhance the process of professional identity formation (see Chapter 1 of this volume). Utilized to its full potential, medical professionals employ reflection as a remarkable tool for deep, lifelong learning, gleaning personal and professional insight and improving clinical skills.

Reflection also provides the groundwork for embedding enhanced approaches to structure, processes, and interactions in medical practice. These approaches are learned through self-rumination and the contemplation of concurrent systems, procedures, and group efforts. Furthermore, a relationship between reflective ability and professionalism has been identified, which supports the incorporation of reflection into the curriculum for clinicians. In this chapter, we will establish the foundational thinking supporting the reflective process and then provide structured frameworks to engage in it.

Reflective practice in healthcare education is an emerging topic with a substantial theoretical basis. In today's complex and ever-changing healthcare environment, clinicians must work to continuously adapt and refresh their knowledge and skills by learning from their experiences. The field has continued to mature, and the benefits of reflective practice continue to be identified, with the concepts and interpretations of reflection drawing from a long history of research in philosophy and education.

Reflection may also potentially play a role in mitigating physician burnout and restoring the voice of physicians. Reflection has a "therapeutic function, particularly for promoting serious self-assessment. Specifically, reflection has been identified in the literature as helping physicians deal with traumatic events, in addition to regenerating their enthusiasm and creativity and providing an opportunity for catharsis."[1p1] With today's epidemic of physician burnout, engaging in reflective thinking may be one of the best things that we can do for ourselves.

Prevailing theories on reflection

Reflection has been discussed in the academic literature since the early 1930s. As our thinking has evolved, there have been dozens of theories presented that have implications in education, social sciences, medicine, law, and other fields. In this section, we will describe five theoretical frameworks of reflection posited by Dewey, Schon, Brookfield, Kolb, and Gibbs; the final two frameworks have special relevance as practical guides for structured reflection in medical education.

Dewey

John Dewey's work on the role of reflection in education laid the foundation for much of the work currently being done on reflection. In his 1933 work, *How We Think: A Restatement of the Relation of Reflective Thinking to the Educative Process*,[2] Dewey stated that there are four modes of thinking: imagination, belief, stream of consciousness, and reflection. Of these four modes of thinking, Dewey noted that reflection is the only one that contributes to learning. Dewey defined reflection as an "active, persistent, and careful consideration of any belief or supposed form of knowledge, in light of the grounds that support it, and the further conclusions to which it tends."[2p6]

Let's break down Dewey's definition. First, reflection is an *active process*. Dewey also stressed that reflection is a deliberate act. Therefore, it requires subjects to examine purposefully their thoughts and actions to gain insight from which learning can take place. Second, reflection is *persistent*. Actively and continually reflecting on past experiences can be challenging and unsettling, but it takes time and focus on learning to benefit from reflective experience. It is not the reflection of a singular event or experience that will suffice to mold process or professionalism, but the culmination of events and challenges over time. Finally, reflection is *careful*. A specific situation must be considered objectively, with all contributing factors analyzed carefully. One must be particularly aware of the potential for intrinsic bias.

Schon

In *The Reflective Practitioner: How Professionals Think in Action*, published in 1984, Donald Schon described two means of reflection: reflection-in-action and reflection-on-action.[3] An example of reflection-in-action is if a physician encounters an unsuspected problem during treatment that requires her or him to reflect on past cases, experience, or processes to develop a fitting solution. Reflection-on-action takes place after the event, for example, during a morbidity and mortality conference, when one reflects on a case that may have taken an unexpected downturn. When reflection happens in the moment (in-action) and leads to successful clinical decision-making, the benefits are obvious. Reflecting after the fact (on-action) may seem unnecessary to some; after all, that specific situation has concluded, and there undoubtedly new problems have arisen to which the physician must attend, leaving little time to stop and think. However, this second leg of reflection is just as crucial, if not more so, for it helps physicians with the process of clinical judgment formation and improves their ability to decide the best course of treatment when time is short and confounding factors abound. Taking time to reflect allows physicians to think from a different perspective when encountering a similar situation in the future. The process of mentally reviewing the complex decision-making process involved in responding to a problematic case helps one to learn from the success or failure of their response.

How are these different types of reflection related to how we learn? In reality, learning achieved by reflection-in-action is very different than by reflection-on-action. By engaging in reflecting-on-action, you are able participate in a deeper level of learning by challenging your previously held thoughts and theories. Reflection-on-action takes time, energy, and focus and doesn't occur intuitively; however, after practicing repeatedly, and over extended periods of time, it becomes more comfortable and automatic.

Brookfield

Stephen Brookfield describes a process of critical reflection in his 1995 book *Becoming a Critically Reflective Teacher*.[4] Originally developed as a framework drawing from critical theory to help educators improve their teaching, this critical reflection framework can be adapted for healthcare practitioners. According to Brookfield, for reflection to be critical, it must focus on uncovering and challenging power dynamics and hegemonic assumptions. We are able to do so by viewing ourselves through four lenses: the lens of self-observation; the lens of our students; the lens of our peers; and the lens of literature. By considering the perspective of ourselves, our students, our colleagues, and drawing from the current literature, we can become aware of how dominant ideologies feed power dynamics in the healthcare setting. According to Brookfield, hegemony is the "process whereby ideas, structures, and actions that benefit a small minority in power are viewed by the majority of people as wholly natural, preordained, and working for their own good."[4p16] Uncovering power dynamics and hegemonic assumptions is particularly crucial in the practice of medicine because the field is so steeped in tradition. As a result, modern healthcare is rife with preconceived ideas, but it is our responsibility to recalibrate our assumptions for the well-being and safety of patients.

Kolb

David Kolb, drawing from the research of Kurt Lewin, conceptualized reflection as a circular process in 1984 when he published his book *Experiential Learning: Experience as the Source of Learning and Development*.[5] Kolb defines learning as "the process whereby knowledge is created through the transformation of experience."[6p26] Within this framework, the process of learning is more important than the outcomes. Through reflective practice, we are able to form new knowledge to shape our future actions.

In Kolb's cycle of experiential learning, a *concrete experience* leads to a *reflective observation* of the experience. This reflective observation leads to an *abstract conceptualization* of the event, through which we can learn from the experience and make conclusions on how to modify our approach when confronted with similar situations. we can *actively experiment* with their conclusions and implement what we've learned. This enhanced process then leads to a new concrete experience followed by more reflection, learning, and experimenting. It's important to note that people cannot learn, reach an abstract conceptualization, or experiment with a new plan without first engaging in reflective observation.

Gibbs

Graham Gibbs expanded upon the framework of Kolb's reflective cycle by developing a six-stage iterative cycle that he published in his 1988 book *Learning by Doing: A Guide to Teaching and Learning Methods*.[7] Figure 2.1 briefly describes the six stages of the Gibbs framework for reflection: description, feelings, evaluation, analysis, conclusion, and action plan. Table 2.1 includes

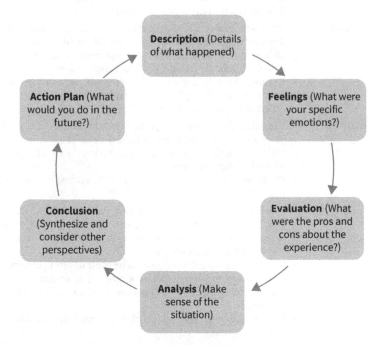

Figure 2.1 Gibbs framework for reflection.

Adapted from G. Gibbs, *Learning by Doing: A Guide to Teaching and Learning Methods* (Oxford: Further Education Unit at Oxford Polytechnic, 1996, online edition 2013). Creative Commons AttributionNonCommercial 3.0 Unported License.

Table 2.1 Gibbs's Framework for Reflection

Stages	Guiding Questions and Suggestions
Stage 1: Description of the event (include as much detail as possible)	• Where were you, and what time of day was it? • Who was there, and who were the primary participants? • Did you play a role, and if so, what was it? • What led up to the event, and what followed? (Think through the entire event, not just the moment that seemed most pivotal.) • What had everyone been doing, and what were their responses?
Stage 2: Feelings and thoughts	• What were you thinking and feeling leading up to the event? • How did the incident affect your emotions and your thought process, both during the event and into the present? • Which people were responsible for causing which emotions? • How do you feel about the outcome of the event? (Try to describe your specific emotions as accurately as possible. If necessary, feeling wheels can be found online and describe emotions in a specific manner. Don't despair if this is difficult at first; we rarely analyze ourselves, especially in writing.)
Stage 3: Evaluation	• Make a judgment about the experience and the outcome. You don't have to definitively decide whether the situation was all bad or all good; in fact, try and find some positives in bad situations and some negatives in good situations. • Expand your thinking about the event and force yourself to view the event through the eyes of others who may have a different impression of the situation.
Stage 4: Analysis	• Consider what you may have read about situations like yours or recall previous, comparable experiences. These components will help you decide what went well during the event and areas of needed improvement. • What did you or others do that led to the success or failure of the venture?
Stage 5: Conclusion	• Synthesize the information you have produced so far: What could you have done differently, and what would you do again? • How could the situation have gone differently if you or others had responded in another way? • Synthesizing the information can be quite different depending on whether you are considering a positive or a negative experience. If the event was positive, can you replicate the outcome? • If it was negative, how can you change your behavior/thoughts/feelings?
Stage 6: Action plan	• What will you do to prepare for and deal with similar experiences in the future? • How will you adapt and change your response?

Adapted from G. Gibbs, *Learning by Doing: A Guide to Teaching and Learning Methods* (Oxford, UK: Further Education Unit at Oxford Polytechnic, 1996, online edition, 2013).

guiding questions that systematically walk the learner through this reflective process. The Gibbs framework is a model of structured reflection in which the stages of the reflective process are clear and easy to follow for both the novice and experienced practitioner. As a result, the Gibbs framework may be well-suited for education of medical professionals.[8]

Professionalization and the reflective process

Reflection reinforces a balanced practice that underscores professionalism and competence through learning and self-assessment. In terms of patient care, reflection provides insight into the dynamics at play in a given situation. It helps physicians examine their inferences and perceptions, as well as the context in an occurrence, episode, or dilemma. Reflective experience promotes a healthy personal disposition and an engaged, patient-centered practice.

For the clinician, reflection has the potential to promote professional identity formation and resilience[9]; it allows personal biases and assumptions to come to light, which can help to clarify and define experiences as well as generate an opportunity for increased sensitivity and respect for themselves, patients, and coworkers. Seasoned professionals benefit from reflection as a tool to bolster and refine communication and performance, engage in self-care, and strengthen leadership qualities.[10] Employing the reflective process is also known to facilitate a reduction in burnout and can mediate the effects of traumatic events.[11]

Working through cognitive dissonance and disequilibrium by engaging in reflection

The theory of cognitive dissonance proposes that one strives for psychological consistency for successful, real-world function. Reflection can, at times, challenge behaviors affected by beliefs and biases, creating inner conflict. The conflict induced by the practice of reflection brings into view opposing beliefs and thought processes.[12] Without proper support, cognitive dissonance can cause mental discord and uneasiness. However, this conflict can also have a constructive role on future thoughts and behaviors.[13] Both

Piaget and Kohlberg recognized that a reaction to disequilibrium was necessary to proceed through development stages.[14] Similarly, the process of professionalization requires one to transition through phases of constructive disequilibrium. By uncovering unfamiliar ideas, values, and perspectives, the reflective process serves to facilitate emotional and cognitive transformations necessary for professional identity formation.

Metacognition

Metacognition refers to the ability to think about one's own cognitive processes; it is the process that gives rise to the reflective process. Advances in neuroscience through the development of functional neuroimaging technologies such as functional magnetic resonance imaging has allowed for the study of basic neural processes. Although the field is still young, a growing number of studies aim to explore the neural bases of reflection and metacognition.[15,16]

The dual process theory is one way of understanding the process of metacognition.[17] According to this theory, there are two types of decision-making processes: Type I and Type II. Type I refers to fast, reflexive decision-making processes based on intuition, whereas Type II refers to analytical decision-making. As physicians, we spend most of our time in the Type I, intuitive mode of decision-making, but this is also where we are most affected by our cognitive biases, potentially leading to clinical errors. By engaging in the analytical process of reflective writing—the Type II mode of thinking—we can train ourselves to uncover our biases and learn from our experiences. In turn, we may develop the neuronal connections necessary to engage in Type I, intuitive decision-making untainted by bias.

Examples of reflective practice in medicine

Recognizing the value of reflective practice, multiple disciplines in medicine have incorporated it into their curricula. For example, medical education that integrates the humanities tends to include reflection. However, the interpretations of the reflective process and need for reflection differ among disciplines. Two examples in which reflective practice is a fundamental component, narrative medicine and team reflection, offer examples of these differences.

Reflection in narrative medicine

Reflection is a critical component of narrative medicine, a field that focuses on treating patients as individuals with unique stories.[18] This field was developed by Rita Charon and colleagues, who recognized the value of *narrative competence*—or the ability to acknowledge, absorb, interpret, and act on the stories and plights of others—in medical practice. By developing narrative competence, physicians can close the gap between themselves and their patients to provide better, more empathic care.

In practice, each patient's narrative of illness is complex and told through words, gestures, silences, and questions. Furthermore, each narrative contains their unique fears and hopes. Arno Kumagai explains that reflecting on illness narratives is unique because it leads to *transformation* within the clinician.[19] This process involves learning on cognitive, affective, and experiential levels and leads toward a perspective that is more open, reflective, and capable of change. For clinicians to uncover the meaning behind patients' narratives and deliver respectful and empathic care, reflective writing can be employed. Drawing from a conceptual model for using creative writing as a process for reflection on patient care and socialization into medicine, narrative medicine incorporates the practice of reflective writing as a tool for developing and practicing narrative competency.[20]

Team reflection

Team reflection supports continued learning, problem-solving, improved patient outcome, and quality improvement initiatives.[21] Interpersonal interactions within teams are most productive when seen as being collaborative, collegial, and where teams possess joint communal values. The automatization of medicine, such as electronic health records and the like, tends to promote interpersonal separation and desocialization. Team reflection offers medical professionals an outlet for collective intelligence and group experience that expands the potentially myopic view of direct individual experience and team-member position. Openness and trust must be the utmost consideration of the team reflection process.

Team reflection encourages the development of psychological safety, defined as "a shared belief held by members of a team that the team is safe for interpersonal risk-taking."[22p354] Psychological safety is revealed in a highly positive work environment that instills feelings of shared initiative and authority, creating an atmosphere where emotions, behaviors, and the nuances of actions and responses of all team members are considered without fear or judgment. This relates to the concept of a high-reliability team that minimizes errors and maximizes patient safety (see Chapter 8 of this volume).[23] Psychological safety thwarts differences in process fulfillment, ideology, and behaviors to unify the team and develop cohesiveness.[24] A benefit to individual team members, psychological safety also bolsters emotional stability and mental health, builds resilience, and supports engagement.[25]

Chapter Quick Summary

- Reflection is a remarkable tool for deep, lifelong learning, gleaning personal and professional insight, and improving clinical skills.
- Reflection provides insight into the dynamics at play in a given situation and examines inferential connotations, perceptions, and context within an occurrence, episode, or dilemma.
- Reflection is an excellent way to bolster and refine communication and performance, allowing for an opportunity for self-care, and can strengthen leadership qualities.
- Reflection can be used to enhance the process of professional identity formation as a tool to work through constructive disequilibrium.
- Five theoretical frameworks of reflection have been posited by Dewey, Schoen, Brookfield, Kolb, and Gibbs.
- Practical models for the reflective process include Gibbs's framework and Kolb's reflective cycle.
- Narrative medicine focuses on treating patients as individuals with their own unique stories, and reflective writing is an important part of developing narrative competency.
- Team reflection supports bases for continued learning, problem-solving, improved patient outcome, and quality improvement initiatives.

Resources

Johnson, H.H., and B.J. Avolio. "Team Psychological Safety and Conflict Trajectories' Effect on Individual's Team Identification and Satisfaction." *Group Organ Manage* 44, no. 5 (2019): 843–873.

Koshy, K., C. Limb, B. Gundogan, K. Whitehurst, and D.J. Jafree. "Reflective Practice in Health Care and How to Reflect Effectively." *Int J Surg Oncol* 2, no. 6 (2017): e20.

McGlinn E.P., and K.C. Chung. "A Pause for Reflection: Incorporating Reflection into Surgical Training." *Ann Plas Surg* 73, no. 2 (2014): 117–120.

Murphy, J.W., B.A. Franz, and C. Schlaerth. "The Role of Reflection in Narrative Medicine." *J Med Educ Curric Dev* 5 (2018): 2382120518785301.

Schrepel, C., J. Jauregui, A. Brown, J. Shandro, and J. Strote. "Navigating Cognitive Dissonance: A Qualitative Content Analysis Exploring Medical Students' Experiences of Moral Distress in the Emergency Department." *AEM Educ Train* 3, no. 4 (2019): 331–339.

WIHI. "How to Navigate Power and Enhance Psychological Safety." February 26, 2020. http://www.ihi.org/resources/Pages/AudioandVideo/how-to-navigate-power-to-enhance-psychological-safety.aspx.

Willcox, G. "The Feeling Wheel: A Tool for Expanding Awareness of Emotions and Increasing Spontaneity and Intimacy." *Transactional Analysis Journal* 12, no. 4 (1982): 274–276. https://doi.org/10.1177/036215378201200411

References

1. Murphy, J.W., B.A. Franz, and C. Schlaerth. "The Role of Reflection in Narrative Medicine." *J Med Educ and Curricular Dev* 5 (2018): 1–5. 2382120518785301.

2. Dewey, J. *How We Think: A Restatement of the Relation of Reflective Thinking to the Educative Process.* Boston: DC Heath, 1910.

3. Schon, D.A. *The Reflective Practitioner: How Professionals Think in Action.* New York: Basic Books, 1984.

4. Brookfield, S.D. *Becoming a Critically Reflective Teacher.* New York: Wiley, 2017.

5. Kolb, D.A. *Experiential Learning: Experience as the Source of Learning and Development.* 1st ed. Englewood Cliffs, NJ: Prentice-Hall, 1984.

6. Wolf, D.M., and D.A. Kolb. "Career Development, Personal Growth and Experiential Learning." In *Organisational Psychology: Readings on Human*

Behaviour. 4th ed. Edited by D.A. Kolb, I.M. Rubin, and J.M. McIntyre. Englewood Cliffs, NJ: Prentice-Hall, 1984.

7. Gibbs, G. *Learning by Doing: A Guide to Teaching and Learning Methods.* Oxford, UK: Further Education Unit, Oxford Polytechnic, Oxford Brookes University, 1988.

8. Husebø, S.E., S. O'Regan, and D. Nestel. "Reflective Practice and Its Role in Simulation." *Clin Simul Nurs* 11, no. 8 (2015): 368–375.

9. Wald, H.S., D. Anthony, T.A. Hutchinson, S. Liben, M. Smilovitch, and A.A. Donato. "Professional Identity Formation in Medical Education for Humanistic, Resilient Physicians: Pedagogic Strategies for Bridging Theory to Practice." *Acad Med* 90, no. 6 (2015): 753–760.

10. Bindels, E., C. Verberg, A. Scherpbier, S. Heeneman, and K. Lombarts. "Reflection Revisited: How Physicians Conceptualize and Experience Reflection in Professional Practice—A Qualitative Study." *BMC Med Educ* 18, no. 1 (2018): 105.

11. Alampi D., and E. Primerano, "Narrative Medicine, Intensive Care and Burn Out." *J Anesth Clin Care* 7 (2020): 48.

12. Horst, A., B.D. Schwartz, J.A. Fisher, N. Michels, and L.J. Van Winkle, "Selecting and Performing Service-Learning in a Team-Based Learning Format Fosters Dissonance, Reflective Capacity, Self-Examination, Bias Mitigation, and Compassionate Behavior in Prospective Medical Students." *Int J Env Res Pub He* 16, no. 20 (2019): 3926.

13. Lewin, R., ed. *The Handbook of Practice and Research in Study Abroad: Higher Education and the Quest for Global Citizenship.* New York: Routledge, 2009.

14. Cruess, R.L., S.R. Cruess, J.D. Boudreau, L. Snell, and Y. Steinert, "A Schematic Representation of the Professional Identity Formation and Socialization of Medical Students and Residents: A Guide for Medical Educators." *Acad Med* 90, no. 6 (2015): 718–725. https://doi.org/10.1097/ACM.0000000000000700

15. Fleming, S.M., and R.J. Dolan. "The Neural Basis of Metacognitive Ability." *Philos T Roy Soc B* 367, no. 1594 (2012): 1338–1349. https://doi.org/10.1098/rstb.2011.0417

16. Molenberghs, P., F.-M. Trautwein, A. Böckler, T. Singer, and P. Kanske. "Neural Correlates of Metacognitive Ability and of Feeling Confident: A Large-Scale fMRI Study." *Soc Cogn Affec Neuro* 11, no. 12 (2016): 1942–1951. https://doi.org/10.1093/scan/nsw093

17. Evans J. St. B.T., and K.E. Stanovich. "Dual-Process Theories of Higher Cognition: Advancing the Debate." *Perspec Psycho Sci* 8, no. 3 (2013): 223–241. https://doi.org/10.1177/1745691612460685

18. Charon, R. "Narrative Medicine: A Model for Empathy, Reflection, Profession, and Trust." *JAMA* 286 (2001): 1897–1902.

19. Kumagai, A.K. "A Conceptual Framework for the Use of Illness Narratives in Medical Education." *Acad Med* 83, no. 7 (2008): 653–658. https://doi.org/10.1097/ACM.0b013e3181782e17

20. Shapiro, J., D. Kasman, and A. Shafer. "Words and Wards: A Model of Reflective Writing and Its Uses in Medical Education." *J Med Human* 27, no. 4 (2006): 231–244. https://doi.org/10.1007/s10912-006-9020-y

21. Ong, Y.H., M.Y.H. Koh, and W.S. Lim. "Shared Leadership in Interprofessional Teams: Beyond Team Characteristics to Team Conditions." *J Interprof Care* 34, no. 4 (2020): 444–452.

22. Edmondson, A. "Psychological Safety and Learning Behavior in Work Teams." *Admin Sci Quart* 44, no. 2 (1999): 350–383.

23. Baker, D.P., R. Day, and E. Salas. "Teamwork as an Essential Component of High-Reliability Organizations." *Health Serv Res* 41, no. 4, pt. 2 (2006): 1576–1598. https://doi.org/10.1111/j.1475-6773.2006.00566.x

24. Rosenbaum, L. 2019. "Cursed by Knowledge: Building a Culture of Psychological Safety." *New Engl J Med* 380, no. 8 (2019): 786–790.

25. Taylor, C., M.F. Dollard, A. Clark, C. Dormann, and A.B. Bakker. "Psychosocial Safety Climate as a Factor in Organisational Resilience: Implications for Worker Psychological Health, Resilience, and Engagement." In *Psychosocial Safety Climate: A New Work Stress Theory*. Edited by M.F. Dollard, C. Dormann, and M.A. Idris, 199–228. New York, Springer, 2019.

3
Happiness and Self-Care

Medical professionalism is not only concerned about patient satisfaction and safety but also with physicians' happiness and satisfaction. Self-care and personal well-being are fundamental tenets of medical professionalism, because physicians ought to care for themselves while attending to their duty to patients and society. Practicing medicine can often be emotionally taxing and challenging. In addition, systemic issues—such as decreases in autonomy and increases in clerical burden—have often been cited as causative factors to unprecedented and widespread levels of physician unhappiness and burnout.[1] Initiatives to identify and address these systemic issues are being studied by many scholars (see Chapter 10 of this volume), as well as clinical depression, physician suicide, and strategies for developing resilience (see Chapters 10 and 11 of this volume).

This chapter will limit its focus on what we individually can do to cultivate happiness and well-being in our personal and professional lives. Many physicians tend to eschew personal happiness, particularly early in their careers, viewing it as something to be obtained in the future. Many of us may remember sacrificing personal time to obtain good grades, study for the MCAT and the board exams, with the belief that we would be happy in the future. We may also recall the lengthy work hours and sleepless nights on-call during residency.

Historically, the culture of medical education and training has espoused the values of hard work and self-sacrifice, often viewing personal happiness as an afterthought. Indeed, we all work hard, and thrive in medicine's quick-paced environment. Is there a place for us to pursue our happiness and to take care of ourselves? We believe that happiness is a state of being that is achievable today, tomorrow, and in the future through incorporating the values of self-care in our daily lives.

This chapter's focus on happiness is not meant to be a one-size-fits-all approach to dictate how you can achieve happiness in your life. Conceptions of happiness are unique to each individual and may change over time.

Nevertheless, we will develop some ideas around different constructs of happiness, and we will introduce some tools that may help you along your path.

Viktor Frankl developed an interesting theory for what makes humans happy. He was held captive in Auschwitz for many years and developed the theory of logotherapy, which posits that the primary motivating factor of human beings is finding meaning in their lives. His book, *Man's Search for Meaning*, describes his and his fellow captives' experiences and how a common thread of finding *meaning* kept them alive even under such horrendous conditions.[2] For example, Frankl notes that thinking of his wife, who was in a different concentration camp, and having imaginary conversations with her, was one of the main factors that kept him alive. Even in a situation in which everything was taken from these prisoners, their ability to shape their attitudes to choose how to respond to their situation remained. Frankl suggests that finding meaning is the key to happiness. As you read this chapter, we suggest that you focus on defining and refining your own sense of purpose and meaning and your personal definition of happiness.

Historical definitions of happiness

So, what is happiness, anyway? Happiness can be an abstract concept and may mean different things to different people. It may be helpful to survey a few of the definitions that have been provided by influential thinkers throughout history. Aristotle believed that happiness was the highest aim of humanity and that it had two main components: *hedonia* (pleasure); and *eudaimonia* (a life well-lived). Hedonia refers to the good feelings experienced when something goes right or when you engage in an activity that you enjoy. Hedonia is a feeling state and may be what people first think of when talking about happiness. However, the concept of eudaimonia, often referred to as *meaning* in contemporary psychology, may be more relevant in our discussion of happiness in the context of medical professionalism.

For the Hellenistic philosophers, the entire purpose of philosophy was to achieve happiness; for Epicurus, this was characterized by *aponia* (an absence of pain). Mahatma Gandhi defined happiness as harmony in what you think, say, and do. Lyubomirsky and colleagues define a happy person as one "who experiences frequent positive emotions, such as joy, interest, and pride, and infrequent (though not absent) negative emotions, such as sadness, anxiety, and anger."[3p816]

When discussing the concept of happiness, the interrelated concept of "well-being" is relevant. Martin Seligman provides a theoretical framework for psychological well-being using the acronym PERMA™.[4] The PERMA™ model states that well-being consists of five main factors:

- *Positive emotions*: Experiencing emotions such as joy, hope, pride, love, gratitude, serenity, interest, amusement, inspiration, and awe.
- *Engagement*: Being completely absorbed in an activity, what positive psychologists call a state of flow.
- *Relationships*: Engaging in positive connections with others.
- *Meaning*: Believing in and serving something that is bigger than yourself.
- *Accomplishments*: Achieving incremental steps toward identified goals.

While PERMA™ was initially developed within the field of positive psychology as a model for assessing patient well-being, it is also useful for evaluating personal happiness. The aim of positive psychology can be summarized as follows: "Treatment is not just fixing what is broken; it is nurturing what is best."[5p7] In Chapter 9 of this volume, we will discuss how positive psychology can be used to improve patient well-being through motivational interviewing and other strategies. In this chapter, we focus on the tangible benefits of personal happiness and ways to develop it. PERMA™ encompasses many of the definitions of happiness provided throughout history, and when we refer to the concept of "happiness" in this book, we equate it with well-being in positive psychology. Happiness is more than just a feeling: it refers to human flourishing and fulfillment.

Happiness: a long-term goal?

Many people state that happiness is their main long-term goal. However, just as the definitions of happiness throughout history differ significantly, people's own conceptions of happiness are unique as well. We suggest that you complete a eulogy exercise to assess what happiness means to you personally (see Box 3.1). In writing a eulogy for your future self, you must

Box 3.1 Write Your Own Eulogy

Imagine after a long, happy, and successful career as a physician and a joyous retirement, you pass away of natural causes. Imagine what your life would have been like. Consider what you would like to be remembered for and take a few minutes to write what comes to mind. Try not to overthink this exercise and avoid overly editing or critiquing your thoughts.

Some guiding questions include

- What was meaningful to you in your life?
- Who did you impact in a positive way?
- What were some of your major accomplishments?
- What were some of your most challenging moments?
- What gave you the most joy?
- What were you passionate about?
- What is your legacy?

evaluate what is most important to you, or how you define happiness. In doing so, you may be better able to actively shape your goals and work toward your idea of happiness.

Responses to Box 3.1 are bound to vary by person. However, your thoughts may help you to identify what is important to you. What were the defining goals, desires, and wishes that you hoped to achieve and would like to be remembered for? Did they involve family? What about the patients you helped? Was getting a final grade of B− in a course one of the items you wrote about in your eulogy? Was every one of your imperfections that seems so huge now displayed in neon lights when you passed away?

As physicians, we are quite proficient in developing treatment plans for our patients. How often would we consider moving forward in treating a patient without first envisioning the steps toward a desired outcome? In the same vein, before moving forward in our own lives, we ought to first develop a plan that encompasses our values, aspirations, and passions.

Measures of happiness

Measuring happiness is often a difficult task, because happiness—often referred to as subjective well-being—is such a subjective concept. However, several self-reported, questionnaire-based measures have been shown to be reliable and valid. These measures assess three main components of happiness: positive affect, absence of negative affect, and life satisfaction. Five of the most common scales are described in Table 3.1.

Biological determinants of happiness

Throughout history, defining happiness has been a largely philosophical question. Recently, through advances in science and technology, studies that assess the biological determinants of happiness have become possible. Much of this work has focused on its hedonic component by measuring the brain's response to reward.[6] Some hedonic mechanisms have been found deep in the brain within ventral striatal circuitry, particularly in the nucleus accumbens and ventral pallidum, and others, in the cortex in the ventral prefrontal region.

While eudaimonic happiness may be more difficult to measure, hedonic and eudaimonic happiness have been found to be highly correlated,[7] and many of the neurological mechanisms implicated in the hedonic experience of sensory pleasure have been found to be active in eudaimonic experiences.[8] Interestingly, though, the patterns of brain activation seem to differ. In a two-year longitudinal study of adolescents, functional magnetic resonance imaging was used to measure the brain's response to two separate tasks that putatively engaged hedonic and eudaimonic happiness, respectively.[9] While both tasks engaged regions of the ventral striatum, the eudaimonic task (a donation task involving personal loss for overall family gain) was correlated with a longitudinal decrease in depressive symptoms, while the hedonic task was not. Therefore, the context in which ventral striatal activation is observed seems to be important and determinative of the networks of neural response.

Resilience, or the ability to recover from negative feelings, has also received significant attention in neuroscience and has been suggested as a key

Table 3.1 Common Scales to Measure Happiness

Name	Developed By	Brief Description
Subjective Happiness Scale	Lyubomirsky and Lepper (1999)[a]	A four-item scale designed to measure subjective happiness. Each item consists of a sentence fragment which can be finished in seven ways. For example, the first question states, "In general, I consider myself," and the answer choices range from "not a very happy person" to "a very happy person."
Oxford Happiness Inventory	Hills and Argyle (2002)[b]	A 29-item questionnaire to assess happiness measured using a six-point Likert scale. Statements include those that are positively scored, such as, "I am intensely interested in other people," and those that are negatively scored, such as, "I am not particularly optimistic about the future."
Positive and Negative Affect Schedule (PANAS) Scales	Watson, Clark, and Tellegen (1988)[c]	A 20-item scale measuring positive and negative affect measured on a 5-point Likert scale. Respondents are asked to indicate how they generally feel emotions such as "interested," "upset," and "enthusiastic."
Satisfaction with Life Scale	Deiner, Emmons, Larsen and Griffin (1985)[d]	A five-item scale designed to measure global cognitive judgments of one's life satisfaction (eudaimonic components of happiness) measured on a seven-point Likert scale. Statements to respond to include, "So far I have gotten the important things I want in life."
Values in Action (VIA) Survey of Character Strengths	Peterson and Seligman (2004)[e]	A 240-item scale measured on a five-point Likert scale designed to measure the degree to which respondents endorse items reflecting the 24-character strengths that comprise the VIA Classification. Statements include "Being able to come up with new and different ideas is one of my strong points."

[a]Lyubomirsky, S., and H.S. Lepper. "A Measure of Subjective Happiness: Preliminary Reliability and Construct Validation." *Soc Ind Res* 46, no. 2 (1999): 137–155. https://doi.org/10.1023/A:1006824100041

[b]Hills, P., and M. Argyle. "The Oxford Happiness Questionnaire: A Compact Scale for the Measurement of Psychological Well-Being." *Pers Indiv Differ* 33, no. 7 (2002): 1073–1082. https://doi.org/10.1016/S0191-8869(01)00213-6

[c]Watson, D., L.A. Clark, and A. Tellegen. "Development and Validation of Brief Measures of Positive and Negative Affect: The PANAS Scales." *J Pers Soc Psychol* 54, no. 6 (1988): 1063–1070. https://doi.org/10.1037//0022-3514.54.6.1063

[d]Diener, E., R.A. Emmons, R.J. Larsen, and S. Griffin. "The Satisfaction with Life Scale." *J Pers Assess* 49, no. 1 (1985): 71–75. https://doi.org/10.1207/s15327752jpa4901_13

[e]Peterson, C., and M.E. Seligman. *Character Strengths and Virtues: A Handbook and Classification.* Vol. 1. New York: Oxford University Press, 1994.

mechanism for sustained happiness.[10] By being able to quickly recover from negative events, one is able to maintain a long-term state of happiness even in the face of adversity. By measuring the recovery time of amygdala activation in subjects following a negative stimulus, researchers have found that participants who scored higher on the Purpose in Life, Personal Growth, and Self-Acceptance subscales of the Six-Factor Model of Psychological Well-Being[11] exhibited the most robust recovery.[12] It has been theorized that connectivity between the prefrontal cortex and amygdala is one key node for mediation of happiness.

Another constituent of happiness with a neural basis is prosocial behavior. The quality of one's social connections is one of the strongest predictors of happiness and well-being.[13] In fact, social isolation activates many of the same brain regions as physical pain.[14] On the other hand, behavior that increases social bonds has been shown to increase well-being.[15-17] A vital precursor to prosocial behavior is empathy, or the ability to recognize and share the emotions of others. Research suggests that the regions of the brain generally implicated in the empathic response include the anterior insula and anterior cingulate cortex. (We will discuss the concept of empathy and the neural basis of different types of empathic responses in further detail in Chapter 6 of this volume.)

Elevated levels of happiness are therefore associated with individuals who experience positive emotions, recover more quickly from negative experiences, and engage in empathic and altruistic acts. Therefore, it seems evident that happiness has multiple neurological components that work in tandem. Crucially, however, each of the neurological pathways involved in these processes exhibit plasticity, suggesting that happiness can be trained in the brain. For example, meditation has been shown to increase frontal lobe activity and induce hemispheric shifts, orienting the brain from the fight-or-flight response to one of increased satisfaction and acceptance.

So, what else determines our happiness? Much of it seems to be genetic. A study on 4,000 sets of twins suggests that 50 percent of satisfaction from life results from an individual's genes;[18] another study suggests that the other 50 percent of happiness is determined from intentional activity (40 percent) and from circumstance (10 percent).[19] Therefore, while happiness does have a significant genetic basis, it is also dependent on an individual's mindset and actions.

While research on neuromodulators and their effects have mostly focused on their implications in disease states, it is evident that happiness is influenced by a complex interaction of neurotransmitters and hormones. These include, but are not limited to dopamine, norepinephrine, gamma-aminobutyric acid, serotonin, oxytocin, and beta-endorphin. Imbalances of these neuromodulators may have widespread effects on mood, thoughts, and feelings. However, brain chemistry can be affected through behavioral change. Mindfulness and meditation have been shown to affect concentrations of gamma-aminobutyric acid in the brain. Exercise has been shown to increase levels of beta-endorphin, while intimate contact has been shown to increase production of oxytocin. Later in this chapter, we will discuss specific strategies that you can use to positively affect happiness.

Pursuing happiness

Over 240 years ago, our nation was founded on the "unalienable Rights... [of] Life, Liberty, and the pursuit of Happiness."[20] One might wonder how far we have come in attaining happiness within our nation. Data from the past 60 years show that, while the average income in the United States has increased, people are no more happier now than they were in the late 1950s.[21] Thus, research supports the common saying that "money can't buy happiness." Furthermore, an analysis of data from more than 1.7 million people in 164 different countries taken from the Gallup World Poll found that maximal satiation for life evaluation occurs at an income level of $95,000 but at $60,000 to $75,000 for emotional well-being.[22]

Although overall wealth has increased, happiness has not, and this can be explained in part by the hedonic treadmill. The hedonic treadmill describes the tendency for people to remain at a relatively stable level of happiness despite major positive events or achievement of goals. Consider the process of buying a new cell phone. After saving money for this phone, you are finally able to purchase it, and you receive a boost of satisfaction. However, after a few weeks, you become used to having a new phone, and you find that you are now rather bored by it. An even newer and more expensive phone model comes out. Instead of being content with the phone you have, you find yourself wanting the new one; then, the treadmill repeats. We constantly seek a higher level of stimulation to maintain a base level of satisfaction.

Behavioral studies with rats support the existence of a hedonic tread-mill: the notion that a more frequent and intense level of stimulation is needed to produce the same level of pleasure.[23] Rats were placed in cages with a lever that, when pressed, activated an electrode that was connected to the lateral hypothalamus of the rat. The electrode triggered the "reward system" of the brain, releasing dopamine and reinforcing the rat's behavior. After the first time the rat pressed the lever and felt the stimulation to its brain's pleasure center, the rat began to press the lever more frequently, at the expense of other vital behaviors necessary to function, such as eating and drinking.

Thus, while the pursuit of happiness drives the increase in economic wealth that is observed as a national trend, this pursuit often times does not lead to people becoming happier. As explained by the hedonic treadmill, even after reaching a milestone, people continue to strive for goals that are harder and harder to achieve.

Self-care

Being a physician means that we experience anxiety and grief when dealing with our patients' suffering. Unchecked, these emotions can lead to empathic distress, which can further lead to disengagement and burnout. In Chapter 6 of this volume, we discuss the different modes of empathic responses and how the cognitive mode of empathic concern, often referred to as compassion, can help abate feelings of distress. However, changes within the paradigms of healthcare have led to unprecedented levels of unhappiness within the physician population, as evidenced by the sobering figures of physician burnout, depression, and suicide.

Although widespread physician unhappiness is largely a systemic problem, and initiatives to combat these issues at policy and institutional levels have begun, perhaps the most effective thing we can do at the individual level as physicians is to engage in self-care. Self-care refers to strategies for individual physicians to take care of themselves and has been gaining traction as a professional imperative. The revised edition of the Declaration of Geneva, published by the World Medical Association in 2017, now includes the clause, "I will attend to my own health, well-being, and abilities in order to provide care of the highest standard."[24] The Charter on Professional Well-Being, published by the Collaborative for Healing and Renewal in Medicine (CHARM), outlines a commitment to raising awareness to both individual and system-level interventions for promoting physician well-being.[25] Self-care begins with the "recognition that people have multiple personal dimensions to attend to in order to live a 'good' life including inner lives, families, work, community, and spirituality."[26p78] This concept of a "good life" that includes all of these factors is similar to our definition of happiness, and therefore self-care can be viewed as a tool to shape personal happiness.

Self-care strategies

Self-care includes actions at both the personal and professional levels. One example of personal self-care is engaging in meditation or mindfulness exercises. Because happiness is in the brain and can be shaped through our thoughts and actions as per the concept of neuroplasticity, meditation and mindfulness are ways to transform our attitudes and perceptions to foster happiness. Mindfulness and meditation have been shown to lead to an increase in gray matter concentration within the left hippocampus, as well as the right insula and the somatosensory cortex, which are involved in learning and memory processes, emotion regulation, self-referential processing, and perspective-taking. These changes may contribute to a decrease in worry, anxiety, and depression.

Making a habit of practicing mindfulness or meditation each day can do wonders for your happiness and mental health (see Exercise 3.2). While some may claim that these exercises are hard to incorporate within our already packed schedules, some of these exercises can be done in just a few minutes. For example, you may choose to close your eyes and listen to your breathing for a few minutes in between seeing patients in the clinic or observe nature with a renewed perspective during a quick walk during a lunch break. Meditation and mindfulness are easy to incorporate into a daily routine and are excellent ways to mitigate the stresses of professional life.

In the past few years, it has become even easier to practice mindfulness and other self-care exercises with the invention of smartphone self-help applications (see Box 3.2). There have only been a few studies that have evaluated their effectiveness, but several studies exploring various mindfulness-training applications found that their use is associated with positive effects on well-being, quality of life, stress, and resilience.[27]

Box 3.2 Practicing Mindfulness

An example of a mindfulness exercise you can practice each day is focusing on your breathing. Sit down in a chair with your back flat, close your eyes, and breathe deeply in and out. Think about the air filling your lungs and then leaving. Let all of your other thoughts fade away. If other thoughts do intrude on your mind space, gently let your mind come back to your breath. After a few minutes, return to normalcy. You'll likely notice that you feel rejuvenated and happier than before.

Another way to practice mindfulness is by observing things in your day-to-day lives with a new perspective. Build a new-found awareness of your surroundings. You'll likely find that many of the objects you encounter each day have details that you have never noticed before. As you become more aware of your surroundings, you may be able to develop a deeper connection with them.

Maintaining a healthy lifestyle through adequate sleep, nutrition, and exercise is also a vital component of self-care. Research shows that lifestyle contributes significantly to well-being. Many physicians may feel that they do not have the time and resources to focus on their health. In a demanding career, lifestyle sometimes stops being a priority. However, some of the most important things you can do for your personal happiness are to sleep and eat well and exercise regularly. (We will discuss these concepts further in Chapter 9 of this volume where we introduce the new evidence-based field of lifestyle medicine.)

Perhaps the most important self-care strategy is developing meaningful connections, both in and outside of the workplace. In an 80-year longitudinal study of happiness at Harvard called the Grant Study, researchers found that the nature of our relationships and our level of happiness in them exerts a profound effect on our health.[28] While taking care of our bodies through healthy lifestyle choices is a vital part of self-care, developing social connections is also crucial for happiness. Experiencing loneliness leads to decreases in happiness, measurable declines in brain function, and earlier death. One landmark study found that lack of social connection is a greater detriment to health than obesity, smoking, and high blood pressure.[29]

However, it is not about the quantity of social connections, but rather about the quality. According to George Vaillant, one of the principle investigators of the Grant Study at Harvard, the warmth of our relationships plays as pivotal role on our life satisfaction. As physicians, many of our most meaningful relationships may be developed in the workplace, with other members of our healthcare team and with trainees. However, taking time to develop meaningful personal relationships outside of the workplace is also vital. Even when we feel pressed for time due to our demanding schedules, making an effort to maintain relationships may result in great benefits in the long run.

Expectation management

Expectation management is an aspect of self-care that may aid in developing happiness. A longitudinal study of 29,000 Americans between ages 18 to 88 between 1972 and 2004 reported that the odds of being happy increase 5 percent with every 10 years of life, with older Americans being the happiest.[30] The authors purport that this is due to the fact that older Americans have learned to lessen their expectations and be more content with their lives. This study also found that baby boomers are the least happy, perhaps because of their achievement-oriented mindset and accompanying struggles with expectation management.

In general, most physicians are aspirational, hard-working, and goal-oriented. Indeed, it is difficult to become a physician without having these qualities. However, to not get stuck in the hedonic treadmill, we must learn to manage expectations and reframe our goals. Hopefully, the eulogy exercise (Box 3.1) provided some insight into your personal idea of happiness. It may be helpful to continually engage in reflection to think about what really matters to you to manage expectations and shape actions.

Final considerations

As a healer, physician, and medical professional, you will be exposed to human suffering daily, even hourly. Holding onto a sense of love, positivity, happiness, and the human capacity for goodness will be challenged. As physicians, we need time to heal; we need to be able to renew our trust and faith in each other. Otherwise, we may get tired and weary. The mental exhaustion we experience is a normal process and understandable when considering the emotional connections we make with our patients and our work. Not having time or giving ourselves time to heal and step away from the pain and suffering that is a part of our patients' experiences can lead to a blunting of affect, distancing from the emotions, and robotic work life. Changes in healthcare are creating an overworked and underrested physician workforce. Until the necessary systemic changes are made to the healthcare system, it is ultimately your responsibility and duty to focus on your mental health. Take the breaks, find joy outside of medicine, and renew your love of life and humankind.

In medicine, you may find yourself thinking that there are an infinite amount of patients whom you must see, problems that you must solve, and new knowledge that you will never be able to learn. You will never be able to know everything there is to know about your profession or be able to help all of the patients who need help. This can often be very frustrating for physicians, but it is important for medical professionals to have realistic expectations for their work. By managing your expectations and taking care of yourself, you can allow yourself to be a happier physician who is ultimately able to be more effective in your job. One of the goals of this book is to help manage your expectations for your profession, increase your happiness, and ultimately give you the tools to help you get through the rough parts of the medical field.

Chapter Quick Summary

- Self-care and personal well-being are fundamental tenets of medical professionalism.
- Happiness is a state of being that is achievable today, tomorrow, and in the future.
- The definition of happiness is individual for each person but can be thought of as consisting of five main factors: positive emotions, engagement, relationships, meaning, and accomplishments.

- Happiness has genetic and environmental determinants.
- The concept of the hedonic treadmill explains why overall happiness tends to remain the same.
- Self-care strategies and expectation management can help us to maintain our happiness.
- Physicians are exposed to human suffering daily and have challenging responsibilities, but we should work to maintain happiness.

Resources

Achor, S. *The Happiness Advantage: The Seven Principles of Positive Psychology that Fuel Success and Performance at Work.* New York: Broadway Books, 2010.

Csikszentmihalyi, M. *Finding Flow: The Psychology of Engagement With Everyday Life.* 2nd ed. New York: Basic Books, 2020.

Gilbert, D. "The Surprising Science of Happiness" [Video]. *TED2004.* February 2004. https://www.ted.com/talks/dan_gilbert_the_surprising_science_of_happiness#t-450830.

"Motivation: Self-Stimulation in Rats" [Video]. Posted December 10, 2010. https://www.youtube.com/watch?v=aNXhyPj-RsM

His Holiness the Dalai Lama and H.C. Cutler. *The Art of Happiness: A Handbook for Living.* New York: Riverhead Books, 2009.

Hoff, B. *The Tao of Pooh.* New York: Dutton, 1982.

Peterson, C. *A Primer in Positive Psychology.* New York: Oxford University Press, 2006.

Ricard, M. *Happiness: A Guide to Developing Life's Most Important Skill.* 2nd ed. Trans. J. Browne. New York: Little Brown, 2016.

Santos, L. "The Science of Well-Being" [Course]. *Yale University.* https://www.coursera.org/learn/the-science-of-well-being

Schwartz, B. *The Paradox of Choice: Why More Is Less.* New York: Ecco Press, 2004.

Seligman, M. *Authentic Happiness: Using the New Positive Psychology to Realize Your Potential for Lasting Fulfillment.* New York: Free Press, 2002.

Via Institute on Character. [Homepage]. https://www.viacharacter.org/

Waldinger, R. What Makes a Good Life? Lessons from the Longest Study on Happiness *TEDxBeaconStreet.* November 2015. https://www.youtube.com/watch?v=8KkKuTCFvzI.

References

1. National Academies of Sciences, Engineering, and Medicine. *Taking Action Against Clinician Burnout: A Systems Approach to Professional Well-Being* Washington, DC: National Academies Press, 2019. http://www.ncbi.nlm.nih. gov/books/NBK552618/

2. Frankl, V.E. *Man's Search for Meaning: An Introduction to Logotherapy.* New York: Simon & Schuster, 1984.

3. Lyubomirsky, S., L. King, and E. Diener. "The Benefits of Frequent Positive Affect: Does Happiness Lead to Success?" *Psychol Bull* 131, no. 6 (2005): 803–855. https://doi.org/10.1037/0033-2909.131.6.803

4. Seligman, M. *Flourish.* New York: Free Press, 2011.

5. Seligman, M.E.P., and M. Csikszentmihalyi. "Positive Psychology: An Introduction." *Am Psychol* 55, no. 1 (2000): 5–14. https://doi.org/10.1037/0003-066X.55.1.5

6. Kringelbach, M.L., and K.C. Berridge. "The Neuroscience of Happiness and Pleasure." *Soc Res* 77, no. 2 (2010): 659–678.

7. Diener, E., P. Kesebir, and R. Lucas. "Benefits of Accounts of Well-Being—For Societies and For Psychological Science." *Appl Psych* 57, no. s1 (2008): 37–53. https://doi.org/10.1111/j.1464-0597.2008.00353.x

8. Berridge, K.C., and M.L. Kringelbach. "Building a Neuroscience of Pleasure and Well-Being." *Psych Well-Being* 1, no. 1 (2011): 1–3. https://doi.org/10.1186/2211-1522-1-3

9. Telzer, E.H., A.J. Fuligni, M.D. Lieberman, and A. Galván. "Neural Sensitivity to Eudaimonic and Hedonic Rewards Differentially Predict Adolescent Depressive Symptoms over Time." *P Natl Acad Sci* 111, no. 18 (2014): 6600–6605. https://doi.org/10.1073/pnas.1323014111

10. Russo, S.J., J.W. Murrough, M.-H. Han, D.S. Charney, and E.J. Nestler. "Neurobiology of Resilience." *Nat Neurosci* 15, no. 11 (2012): 1475–1484. https://doi.org/10.1038/nn.3234

11. Ryff, C.D. "Happiness Is Everything, or Is It? Explorations on the Meaning of Psychological Well-Being." *J Pers Soc Psych* 57, no. 6 (1989): 1069–1081.

12. Schaefer, S.M., J. Morozink Boylan, C.M. van Reekum, R.C. Lapate, C.J. Norris, C.D. Ryff, and R.J. Davidson. "Purpose in Life Predicts Better Emotional Recovery from Negative Stimuli." *PloS One* 8, no. 11 (2013): e80329. https://doi.org/10.1371/journal. pone.0080329

13. Diener, E., and M.E.P. Seligman. "Very Happy People." *Psych Sci* 13, no. 1 (2002): 81–84. https://doi.org/10.1111/1467-9280.00415

14. Eisenberger, N.I. "The Pain of Social Disconnection: Examining the Shared Neural Underpinnings of Physical and Social Pain. *Nat Rev Neurosci* 13, no. 6 (2012): 421–434. https://doi.org/10.1038/nrn3231

15. Aknin, L.B., J.K. Hamlin, and E.W. Dunn. "Giving Leads to Happiness in Young Children." *PloS One* 7, no. 6 (2012): e39211. https://doi.org/10.1371/journal.pone.0039211

16. Dunn, E.W., L.B. Aknin, and M.I. Norton. "Spending Money on Others Promotes Happiness." *Science* 319, no. 5870 (2008): 1687–1688. https://doi.org/10.1126/science.1150952

17. Aknin, L.B., C.P. Barrington-Leigh, E.W. Dunn, J.F. Helliwell, J. Burns, R. Biswas-Diener, I. Kemeza, P. Nyende, C.E. Ashton-James, and M.I. Norton. "Prosocial Spending and Well-Being: Cross-Cultural Evidence for a Psychological Universal." *J Pers Soc Psych* 104, no. 4 (2013): 635–652. https://doi.org/10.1037/a0031578

18. Lykken, D., and A. Tellegen. "Happiness Is a Stochastic Phenomenon." *Psych Sci* 7, no. 3 (1996): 186–189. https://doi.org/10.1111/j.1467-9280.1996.tb00355.x

19. Lyubomirsky, S., K.M. Sheldon, and D. Schkade. "Pursuing Happiness: The Architecture of Sustainable Change." *Rev Gen Psychol* 9, no. 2 (2005): 111–131.

20. "Declaration of Independence: A Transcription (July 4, 1776)." *National Archives.* July 20, 2020. https://www.archives.gov/founding-docs/declaration-transcript

21. Laitman, M. "The Study of Happiness." *The Wisdom of Kabbalah.* 2014. http://www.kabbalah.info/eng/content/view/frame/108901?/eng/content/view/full/108901&main

22. Jebb, A.T., L. Tay, E. Diener, and S. Oishi. "Happiness, Income Satiation and Turning Points around the World." *Nat Hum Behav* 2, nos. 33–38 (2018). https://doi.org/10.1038/s41562-017-0277-0

23. Olds, J., and P. Milner. "Positive Reinforcement Produced by Electrical Stimulation of Septal Area and Other Regions of Rat Brain." *J Comp Physiol Psych* 47, no. 6 (1954): 419–427. https://doi.org/10.1037/h0058775

24. Parsa-Parsi, R.W. "The Revised Declaration of Geneva: A Modern-Day Physician's Pledge." *JAMA* 318, no. 20 (2017): 1971–1972. https://doi.org/10.1001/jama.2017.16230

25. Thomas, L.R., J.A. Ripp, and C.P. West. "Charter on Physician Well-Being." *JAMA* 319, no. 15 (April 17, 2018): 1541–1542. https://doi.org/10.1001/jama.2018.1331

26. Sanchez-Reilly, S., L.J. Morrison, E. Carey, R. Bernacki, L. O'Neill, J. Kapo, V.S. Periyakoil, and J. deLima Thomas. "Caring for Oneself to Care for Others: Physicians and Their Self-Care." *J Support Oncol* 11, no. 2 (2013): 75–81.

27. Howells, A., I. Ivtzan, and F.J. Eiroa-Orosa. "Putting the 'App' in Happiness: A Randomised Controlled Trial of a Smartphone-Based Mindfulness Intervention to Enhance Wellbeing." *J Happiness Stud* 17, no. 1 (2016): 163–185. https://doi.org/10.1007/s10902-014-9589-1

28. Vaillant, G. E. *Triumphs of Experience: The Men of the Harvard Grant Study.* Cambridge, MA: Harvard University Press, 2012. https://doi.org/10.4159/harvard.9780674067424

29. House, J.S., K.R. Landis, and D. Umberson. "Social Relationships and Health." *Science* 241, no. 4865 (1988): 540–545. https://doi.org/10.1126/science.3399889.

30. Yang, Y. "Social Inequalities in Happiness in the United States, 1972 to 2004: An Age-Period-Cohort Analysis." *Am Sociol Rev* 73, no. 2 (2008): 204–226.

4
Artificial Intelligence in Medicine

The term "artificial intelligence" (AI) was originally conceived by John McCarthy.[1] The field of AI in medicine first surfaced in the 1970s[2] but has gained significant traction recently due to advances in computing power, data storage, and even algorithmic power. AI is a technological system designed to perform tasks that are commonly associated with human intelligence and ability. The term is associated with tasks that we consider to be fundamentally human that include having the capability to reason, the ability to learn from past experiences, and having the necessary computational power to generate meaning.[3] Early research in AI focused on problem-solving and the capacity to mimic extremely basic human reasoning. Often done by the U.S. Department of Defense, this research paved the way for automation and mimicked higher levels of human reasoning as we see in various computational models today.

AI can be categorized as either *applied* or *generalized*. Applied AI, also referred to as *narrow AI*, utilizes a highly specialized operational system that can simulate and often surpass human capability for vastly distinctive and specific purposes. Applied AI is used frequently to further progress and efficacy in the financial, commercial, manufacturing, and even consumer sectors. In the financial sector, applied AI aids in detecting fraudulent credit card use, while in the commercial sector, it is used to recommend products based on search history. In the manufacturing sector, applied AI is used to predict errors pre-emptively and to manage the production process, and in the consumer sector, it performs in the development of automated assistants like Siri and the development of self-driving cars.

The possibilities for the use of applied AI applications in the medical field are endless. Other than being used as a diagnostic tool, AI is also being used to make physicians' jobs easier. Many physicians use speech-recognition technology as a tool for medical dictation. In the future, AI could also be used to listen to patient consultations and summarize them automatically. This would reduce the time that physicians need to spend on typing electronic health records, allowing them to focus on other tasks that require their attention. Eventually, AI could assess patients' needs by analyzing language, physical gestures, and social signals to detect psychological distress in patients.[4]

In contrast to the direct measures of applied AI, generalized AI is far more interactive with the processes and outcomes it effectuates. Generalized AI is far more controversial and has been slower to gain traction because it requires much more sophisticated computer processes and innovational leaps. Fully accomplished generalized AI is the long-term ambition for science, the actualized wave of the future. For generalized AI to interact with the world, an extremely high amount of processing power is needed to mimic the human brain, and a more fundamental understanding of this organ and its internal interactions is necessary. Currently, generalized AI is working to create processes that can learn.

Disruptive innovation

AI is an example of *disruptive innovation* in healthcare.[5] The descriptive term "disruptive innovation" was coined by Clayton Christensen to describe situations when a small business with a new concept or product disrupts the schema, operational process, or production of an existing industry. Disruption innovation, therefore, is a major change, an innovation that transforms. While disruption may cause upheaval, temporary disorder, a little turbulence, and maybe even an uproar, it is progress at its finest. One's ability to adapt to the disruption most often determines how a person perceives it.

To lend historical context to the idea of disruptive forces, let's analyze an example from our everyday world. When the postal service was first created, it was an important advancement in the history of the United States. People could communicate efficiently and relatively quickly with each other across great distances. If we fast forward several hundred years to the present day, postal mail is now considered to be "snail mail" because it doesn't arrive instantaneously like email does. What is interesting about this change is how rapidly it occurred and how it seemingly came from left field. This example highlights how disruptive forces (e.g., the creation of the internet) can render old traditions, practices and, in this case, technologies relatively useless.

The same trend is expected to occur for AI. Opponents of this new technology believe the potential for AI to make a significant impact on the healthcare field is minimal; however, disruptive forces like AI will continue to impact the world and the field of medicine as we know it.

Historical trends in healthcare

The healthcare industry has traversed, adapted, and thrived through significant changes in its long history. The development of vaccinations, antibiotics, and the concept of sterilization have impacted the lives of all of us, and future innovations will continue to leave their mark.

In addition to changes driven by innovative technologies, *care focus* is transforming the healthcare world. By care focus, we mean the degree to which products, appointments, and procedures cater to either hospitals or patients. Currently, healthcare is in the midst of a transition from hospital-based care to patient-centered care. More and more, so many patients rely on technology to provide health information that healthcare is moving toward preventative and outpatient-centric care. Current examples of technology that we take for granted include home blood pressure monitors, smartwatches, and mobile glucose monitors that have made many in-hospital devices obsolete. The ability to check for a temperature at home changed the point-of-care treatment options many years ago. As such, healthcare is an industry primed for disruptive innovation in the technological sector.

The number of stakeholders in healthcare is extremely high, which leads to more economic capital for innovation. This makes the healthcare industry an ideal place for AI to establish a strong foothold. AI is highly complex, yet it can simplify the processes on which practitioners base their care and treatment of patients. AI's intricate nature requires an understanding of its terms and capabilities relative to the broader technological system.

Machine learning

Machine learning is a subset of AI. It focuses on using statistical techniques to build intelligent computer systems to learn from databases available to it. The key part of machine learning is its ability to learn from data, so it does not require human intervention to change its algorithm. Therefore, machine learning is dynamic and can become more efficient and more accurate than its original algorithm, which was programmed by humans.

Typical uses of machine learning include face detection in an image, speech recognition systems, Spotify suggesting songs to regular users, and many other predictive algorithms. Machine learning could be useful in treating patients with chronic conditions. In healthcare, 50 percent of the total costs come from 5 percent of total patients with these chronic conditions, and those requiring consistent, constant care has gradually increased across the country. Machine learning can be used to identify patients who may be more prone to recurring illnesses, recognize patterns within DNA to find mutations and predict genetic changes, detect anomalies during image processing at a much faster rate and with a higher degree of accuracy, provide effective precision treatments in less time, and assist with the diagnosis of diseases.

In the future, machine learning will recommend the best medications for patients based on their electronic health record. For example, when physicians attempt to create a treatment plan for patients, they will use AI to review treatment options, evaluate the patient's current medication list, check for interactions, and choose the most appropriate combination of drugs for each person.[6] With enough data from humans, a patient's electronic health record could also become a reliable risk predictor for various diseases. AI could also include new personal devices and wearables that could monitor a person's general health. For example, digestible microchips could alert physicians if patients stop taking their medications.[7]

Deep learning

Deep learning is a subset of the field of machine learning and is one of the most recent and advanced developments in AI. Deep learning was inspired by looking at the way our brains function. The algorithms involved in deep learning are called artificial neural networks; these have several different processing layers that all contribute to learning from data.

Deep learning can be difficult to conceptualize, but it may be easier to understand if we use an example. AlphaZero is a computer program developed by the AI research company DeepMind. On December 5, 2017, DeepMind launched a pre-edition of AlphaZero that learned how to play chess completely on its own after only being programmed with the basic rules of the game. There was no strategy introduced to the computer at all, but AlphaZero mastered the game after spending only nine hours learning its strategy by playing against itself and collecting data from these games. It was able to beat traditional chess engines such as Stockfish and Deep Blue, which rely on thousands of rules and heuristics that were created by the best human chess players.[8] Instead of relying on heuristics, AlphaZero has a deep neural network that learns through reinforcement. Because AlphaZero was self-taught, it created many of its inventive strategies for how to play chess that humans had not used before.[10]

The example of AlphaZero and deep learning is very different from earlier examples of AI, such as IBM's computer Deep Blue. Deep Blue was programmed with general strategies of the game of chess and decided on moves by calculating the probability of success for each possibility. Deep Blue first played a six-game chess match against the reigning chess champion, Gary Kasparov, on February 10, 1996 and lost 4 to 2. After upgrades to the computer, a rematch held in May of 1997 was won by Deep Blue with a score of 3.5 to 2.5. Rather than only calculating probabilities, deep learning is creative AI that can learn from itself instead of relying on programming from humans.

Currently, healthcare implements generalized AI in a variety of ways. For example, an initiative based out of Germany has developed a deep learning convolutional neural network to diagnose melanoma more accurately than most dermatologists.[9] An artificial arrangement of nerves that mimic the processes of the brain as it processes data taken in from the eyes was created. It was trained with over 100,000 pictures of melanomas and missed fewer diagnoses than most dermatologists. This result means it was more sensitive than modern physicians, on average, and had higher specificity (fewer false positives).[4]

Another technology, Enlitic, can detect lung cancer nodules in computed tomography images more accurately than an expert panel of radiologists.[10] When AI is used as a visual diagnostic tool, it has been shown to help physicians in radiology, but it can also aid physicians in pathology and dermatology when identifying rashes. In addition to being used as a visual diagnostic tool, Babylon Health, a digital healthcare startup, is developing AI that has done better than physicians on an exam that general practitioners take in England to test their ability to diagnose.[11] Box 4.1 lists some AI breakthroughs over the years.

Box 4.1 AI Breakthroughs

- 1966: Machine learning provides a response to Polanyi's paradox, the theory that human knowledge and capability are largely beyond our explicit understanding.[12]
- 1997: IBM's Deep Blue beats Chess Grandmaster Kasparov.
- 2011: IBM's Watson defeats the two greatest Jeopardy champions.
- 2016: AlphaGo beats Lee-Se-Dol at the game of Go to win the Google DeepMind Challenge Series.
- 2017: Chinese robot "Dentist" fits implants into the mouth of a patient without human assistance.

Blockchain technology

Blockchain technology is not a type of AI, but is a recently developed system that can be used along with AI to disrupt the way that our world works. A blockchain is a data structure that creates digital ledgers for data. It creates a permanent, time-stamped record of digital events between networks or various parties. Blockchain was originally used in Bitcoin, a type of digital currency, as a way of verifying transactions. However, it could also benefit clinicians and the healthcare system greatly.

One area where blockchain can likely help patients and physicians is with the interoperability of health data and electronic health records. The new technology could store a patient's entire record in one place rather than a patient having different medical records in different hospitals. Blockchain could create a connected healthcare ecosystem, where it is much easier for physicians to communicate with one another and with their patients. This correlative system could save physicians precious time while also reducing the risk of mistakes caused by human error when exchanging clinical data. Having patients' medical records in one place also gives them more autonomy and control over their health data. Blockchain may also be used in precision medicine, cybersecurity, and value-based care and reimbursement. Overall, blockchain is likely to streamline medical practice and create a more efficient and productive workflow.

Economic issues

Major players in the healthcare industry include large hospital systems, insurance companies, physicians, caregivers, and, most importantly, patients. With so many individuals having skin in the game, the economic landscape and the future of the industry is extremely complex and variable. Healthcare is an industry currently characterized by rapid growth and transformation. Russell Reynolds and Associates forecast that global healthcare costs—currently estimated at $6 trillion to $7 trillion per year—will reach more than $12 trillion within just seven years.[13] This extreme increase in healthcare costs parallels expenditures topping $3 trillion in the United States, representing a whopping 17 percent of our gross domestic product (GDP). These costs are rising at almost double the rate of economic growth, which tells us that these rising costs cannot be attributed solely to raw growth in the economy (see Box 4.2).[11]

The federal government distributes more and more funding into programs like Medicare and Medicaid as costs increase. *The Tax Policy Briefing Book* by the Urban-Brookings Tax Policy Center reports that the "federal government spent nearly $1.1 trillion on healthcare in fiscal year 2018. Of that, Medicare claimed roughly $583 billion, Medicaid and the Children's Health Insurance Program (CHIP) about $399 billion, and veterans' medical care about $70 billion." [14] These statistics highlight a fundamental flaw in the status quo: a clear and distinct disparity exists between the affordability of healthcare and the necessity of receiving care. Consumers often do not have the capital to meet these expenditures and thus rely on the federal government to subsidize these increasing healthcare costs.

As the cost of healthcare further spirals out of control, a waterfall-like effect is observed. Patient–physician communication, procedure availability, and even the availability of specialists are impeded, in part, by the increase in cost. As costs increase, physicians are urged, if not required, to see more patients in less time. This could contribute to a sharp decline in the patient–physician relationship, a crucial aspect of medical care. The interaction between physicians and their patients determines the latter's satisfaction with the care provided, their tendency to schedule follow-up appointments and tests, and even medication adherence.[15]

While a number of avenues have been utilized in an attempt to solve these issues with healthcare, the most promising solutions are innovative

Box 4.2 Projected National Health Expenditures, 2018–2027

- Under current law, national health spending is projected to grow at an average rate of 5.5 percent per year for 2018 to 2027 and to reach nearly $6 trillion by 2027.
- Health spending is projected to grow 0.8 percentage point faster than GDP per year over the 2018 to 2027 period; as a result, the health share of GDP is expected to rise from 17.9 percent in 2017 to 19.4 percent by 2027.
- Key economic and demographic factors that are unique to the health-care sector are anticipated to be the major drivers of this growth during 2018 to 2027.
- Prices for healthcare goods and services are projected to grow somewhat faster over 2018 to 2027 (2.5 percent compared to 1.1 percent for 2014 to 2017).
- As a result of comparatively higher projected enrollment growth, average annual spending growth in Medicare (7.4 percent) is expected to exceed that of Medicaid (5.5 percent) and private health insurance (4.8 percent).
- The growth in Medicare enrollment is the key reason that the share of healthcare spending by federal, state, and local governments is expected to increase by 2 percentage points over this period, reaching 47 percent by 2027.
- The insured share of the population is expected to remain stable at around 90 percent throughout 2018 to 2027.

Source: National Health Expenditure Data: Projected. CMS.gov. https://www.cms.gov/Research-Statistics-Data-and-Systems/Statistics-Trends-and-Reports/NationalHealthExpendData/NationalHealthAccountsProjected.html

technologies with AI and machine learning at their core. To provide efficient, effective, and impactful care to patients, physicians can use AI as a tool to help them save time throughout the day. This helps physicians establish meaningful relationships with patients as healthcare costs and the number of patients continue to rise.

   Disruptions to an economy or a way of life due to technology are generally helpful to society in the long run. Our quality of life, extreme poverty rate, literacy rate, average life expectancy, and the child mortality rate have all improved radically in the past 50 years. There is no doubt that our population is better off because of technology and innovation. However, along with new technology comes changes to the workforce that often leave some people unemployed or forced to change professions. To adapt to new technology that has proved to be more efficient than humans, job descriptions, positions, and career paths change in ways that no one would have expected. These changes can sometimes leave people unsatisfied with their new roles and work expectations; however, if people have the resources and the ability to adapt and learn throughout their lives, they tend to be better off. Even when jobs are eliminated by technology, new positions and previously inconceivable new niches in the workforce and industry arise.

   When thinking about technology affecting our economy, there is no need to ask if it will ravage the workforce or create new jobs, because the answer to both questions is yes, it will. The main things that need to be considered include whether the creation of new jobs will offset the destruction of others, the relative speed with which this will occur, and how people will be able to adapt to the new job market if the skills required for these jobs do not match those for which they were previously trained.

   Economists disagree on how exactly AI will affect the job market. Some believe that with the technology we currently have available, almost half of the work that people do could be automated.[16] Others have reported that they think only 9 percent of jobs are currently automatable.[17] A 2016 McKinsey Quarterly report states that less than 5 percent of occupations could be completely automated with our current technology, but almost every occupation could be partially automated, and approximately 60 percent of jobs have over 30 percent of activities that could be automated.[18] Healthcare is a humanistic occupation, but it is estimated that the automation potential of healthcare is around 36 percent.[15] Scientific researchers disagree on the exact number, but as technology develops in the coming years, the potential for automation will only increase. We need to be able to work with technology and be prepared to adapt to the changing field of medicine.

   Currently, physicians are some of the highest paid professionals but may not realize the same earning capacity in the future if they do not respond to changes effectuated by AI. AI will affect all professions' value to society, so how can physicians remain necessary to society so that we can keep our jobs? Today's successful physicians need to have deep knowledge of the hard sciences, but this may not be as important in the future. Therefore, we need to develop skills that work with AI, as well as talents that AI systems cannot perform, such as proficiencies in interpersonal communication, information management, and team management.

AI and machine learning in healthcare

Recently, innovative advances in the amount of data that analysts can collect and interpret have paved the way for AI and machine learning to take root in the healthcare industry. Some issues facing medical professionals can be characterized as data problems. We deal with millions of data points of both structured and numerical data. Structured data like blood pressure and heart rate can easily be assimilated by AI, but unstructured data, such as clinical notes, patient history, and discharge summaries, are another matter. When visiting the doctor, notes are taken on patient health including symptoms, any diagnosis, and actions taken. Unstructured data, ripe with essential information, is difficult to analyze in terms of applying machine learning and AI technology. Relaying unstructured data is problematic due to the "narrative" aspect of medicine. For example, two patients presenting with the same cold will describe their condition in drastically different ways. Additionally, physician notes reflect the doctor's previous experience, background, and training.

The ability to obtain valuable information from unstructured data will prove to be extremely vital in the upcoming years. As we face issues with antibiotic-resistant bacteria, potent viral strains, and chronic disease, gathering insight from thousands of patients can help to prioritize treatment options and elevate care. The more data points gathered and interpreted, the more treatments can be designed to cater to certain conditions and disease manifestations. The combination of machine learning and AI is at the forefront of the data revolution that is facing healthcare today.

The future of healthcare and AI

While some critics of AI are steadfast in their viewpoint that modern technologies can never fully replace the physician, other experts feel that, as technological innovation increases over time, the occupation of the doctor will slowly begin to atrophy. These differing assumptions connect back to the example of the snail mail versus email; although unimaginable, disruptive forces have and will continue to shape the world as we know it. Moshe Vardi argues that machines will eventually become integrated into every major industry in the world today.[19] He believes that, in the future, work will be completely dependent upon machines.[20] The role of the human, Vardi believes, is going to atrophy until only highly specialized jobs are left unaffected. While it is unlikely that AI will replace the physician in coming years, the possibility of machines doing so in the future cannot be ruled out.

Although AI is not at a stage to replace the physician, some aspects of AI have been proven to be more effective, productive, and accurate than that of physicians. The foundation of the medical profession relies on identifying complex patterns and trends. When a doctor notices that a patient has a fever and vomiting, she or he will mentally take these two data points and draw upon their previous experience and training to determine the cause for these symptoms. Technology is inherently better and more efficient at parsing through data points and identifying trends as compared to humans. However, it is also the depth and thoroughness of the data transmitted that will provide a more accurate and appropriate diagnosis or treatment protocol.

Fortunately, AI can also be a tool to help physicians in a way that will alleviate some of the burdens currently placed on them. There are many issues with how our healthcare system is set up, and physicians often experience burnout because of the increased time required spent on maintaining electronic health records and clerical work. AI technologies have the potential to provide supplemental and other types of care as they develop in the future, taking away some of these duties from doctors and nurses. Time will tell how integrated these technologies will be in medicine. However, one thing is certain: AI will have a growing role in medicine, although the extent of its integration will vary.

The future of medical education

The Accreditation Council for Graduate Medical Education (ACGME) first presented a list of physician core competencies in 1999 to identify foundational skills physicians should possess (see Box 4.3). These six competencies were assigned to define and shape medical education. ACGME's intent was to construct learning programs that reflected the skill sets and attributes relevant to the practice of medicine. These core competencies have been adopted into the Maintenance of Certification program by the American Board of Medical Specialties.

The ACGME core competencies continue to represent the aims of the medical profession, but *how* medical professionals achieve them needs revision. Although the amount of medical information today exceeds the scope of the retention capacity of the human mind, medical education still focuses on the acquisition of information and associated applications. Rather than information acquisition through rote learning and memorization, education should prepare physicians through cultivating competencies related to the *management* of information, including working with big data, integrating and collaborating with AI, quality improvement, care coordination, interdisciplinary team building, and team management.

The rise of internet-based medical information creates an atmosphere in which patients feel that they have a competent understanding of health concerns. They therefore feel that they merit a higher level of respect, demand to be informed, are more mindful in their decision-making, and want to be in control over their healthcare. In response to this information-rich environment, medical education should include training in communication that

---

Box 4.3 The Six ACGME Core Competencies

- Practice-based learning and improvement
- Patient care and procedural skills
- Systems-based practice
- Medical knowledge
- Interpersonal and communication skills
- Professionalism

Adapted from the ACGME 1999 Annual Report. https://www.acgme.org/Portals/0/PDFs/an_1999AnnRep.pdf. Used by permission of ACGME.

underscores how to effectively impart essential facts, treatment options, and instructions to patients, with an awareness of how individual bias and values often influence what the patient believes or how they process the information. However, educational programs must also teach students how to dispel misinformation and alleviate the fears of patients tactfully. When confronted with irrelevant and misguided data, the medical professional must realize that the foibles of, and susceptibilities to, erroneous online data are persistent and, therefore, allay patient claims and theories decisively, yet graciously.

Several specific competencies and skills that physicians need in the current healthcare landscape have been described in the literature. These skill sets have been adapted and summarized in Box 4.4.

Needed changes in medical curricula

Statistics, probability, and data analytics are necessary when working with AI, especially with the trend toward precision or *personalized medicine*. As more practitioners and hospitals use AI to support clinical decisions, there will be an increased need for medical professionals who are highly skilled in the science of mathematics, going well beyond the current requirements. In addition to data analysis and mathematical specialization, the required general studies of behavioral science must expand to include additional credit hours in the humanities and social science. Communication studies should also be made a requirement and should include specific team-based and peer-based studies in addition to the critical processes of personal human communication and communicative behaviors.

The need for reform of the standard medical curriculum will not be easy. In Wartman's view, currently change "has been incremental, reactive, and mostly around the margins."[21p149] However, he adds, "Changes in 21st-century medical education must be radical, not incremental."[21p149] Qualifying the needs of the medical profession and a call to action to amend the licensing and accreditation framework is perhaps the best way to begin reorganizing medical education as it will respond to mandated requirements.

Box 4.4 Needed Physician Competencies and Skills

- Leadership skills
- Team approach to healthcare
- Soft skills, such as bedside manner, patient communication, attitude, and the ability to appropriately answer questions
- Psychosocial responsibility in the care of patients
- Strong sense of values and ethics
- Lifelong learning skills
- Research skills
- Cost-effective care: understanding the healthcare system, costs, and economics
- Skills for quality improvement and innovation: we need to be comfortable with technology, data, and analytics, in how to use medical data in our IT systems to improve our care, and digital medicine
- High degree of adaptability
- Maintain trust and support from the community

Adapted from S.A. Wartman and C.D. Combs, "Reimagining Medical Education in the Age of AI," *AMA Journal of Ethics*, 21, no. 2 (2019): E146-E152, https://doi.org/10.1001/amajethics.2019.146. Used by permission.

Developing a professional identity based on disruptive forces in the world

Technology is impacting healthcare, but this should only encourage the medical professional to take a different approach with professional goals, be open to change, and be willing to accommodate technology.

AI offers an opportunity for reliable, standardized health management for the population. Early detection, medication tracking, and streamlined case management will help to make huge strides in patient outcomes and safety, accessibility, and efficiency; informed decision-making; time management; cost reductions; and quality improvement. So, where does that leave the medical professional?

Modern medicine has evolved to the point where today's clinicians simply cannot pull from their memory the abundance of data required—including symptoms, diseases, disorders, physiological anomalies, genetic markers, and other information—to process any and every potential medical case that they may encounter. Machine learning and AI makes possible a wide range of data functions that outperform human capability in terms of sheer *volume*, using a *variety* of information and simulations with incomparable *velocity* and *veracity*. These *four Vs* of big data will augment, if not replace, traditional analytical proficiencies performed by the physician.[22]

Medical practitioners will still need to build clinical knowledge of fundamental elements of medical science, including cell biology, biochemistry, physiology, pathology, and pharmacology. They will also need to be able to interpret statistics and have a deep understanding of human biology and research. However, most medical professionals must be willing to abandon any notion that they are an independent practitioner. The job description of all medical professionals will intrinsically evolve into that of a team player and, effectively, a team manager. In this way, clinicians will always be a key component of a healthcare team of medical professionals that will care for patients with a coordinated, multidisciplinary approach that encompasses all aspects of patient-centered care. Medical professionals will manage diagnostics, therapeutic intervention, preventative medicine, safety, and privacy issues. They will manage and analyze data (see Chapter 8 of this volume).

Medical professionals will need to adapt to data-rich conditions that will necessitate a capacity to glean vital information from and respond to the wealth of information provided. Not only will they need to understand and process the statistics, measurements, and conclusions offered, but they then must use that data in their decision-making and when they articulate findings to the patient. They should embrace the idea of being lifelong learners and the ability to adapt to various situations, including a focus on working with AI and incorporating knowledge-management skills.

Most important is the development of skills such as communication, empathy, and compassion, as these will not be able to be replicated by machines. While it is true that patients visit their doctors for a diagnosis and treatment, they also want a personal relationship, communication, and empathy from their physician (see Chapter 6 of this volume). Without proper communication from physicians, there will be higher utilization rates for diagnostic tests, hospitalizations, and prescriptions. However, when patients perceive empathy from their physician, they are more satisfied and are more likely to comply with what they were told to do, which leads to better outcomes and lower medical costs overall.[12]

Chapter Quick Summary

- AI can be categorized as either applied (for a specific task, such as playing chess or diagnosing melanoma) or generalized (replicating the operation of the human brain).
- AI has automated tasks commonly performed by intelligent beings.
- Machine learning is dynamic and can become more efficient and more accurate than its original algorithm, which was programmed by humans.
- Deep learning involves the use of artificial neural networks that delve into several layers of data that contributes to a deeper level of learning, allowing for fully integrated and accurate results.
- Blockchain technology could store all of patients' records in one place and create a connected health ecosystem.
- Technology will have a major impact on our economy, ravaging the workforce but also creating new jobs.
- There will always be a need for what humans do best: empathy, care, and compassionate understanding.
- AI and other advances in technology require that medical education change its focus and core competencies.

Resources

"AI vs. Doctors: Artificial Intelligence is Challenging Doctors on Their Home Turf. We're Keeping Score." *IEEE Spectrum*. 2020. https://spectrum.ieee.org/static/ai-vs-doctors

AlphaGo. [Homepage]. *DeepMind*. https://deepmind.com/research/alphago/

"Artificial Intelligence in Health Care: Within Touching Distance. *Lancet* 390, no. 10114 (2018): 2739.

Armendariz, A. "What Lies Ahead for the USPS with the Continued Declines in Mail Volume and Revenue? Mailing Systems Technology." *Mailing Systems Technology*.

December 26, 2017. http://mailingsystemstechnology.com/article-4287-What-Lies-Ahead-for-the-USPS-with-the-Continued-Declines-in-Mail-Volume-and-Revenue.html

"Big Data: What It Is and Why It Matters." https://www.sas.com/en_us/insights/big-data/what-is-big-data.html

Bresnick, J. "Top 12 Ways Artificial Intelligence Will Impact Health Care." *HealthITAnalytics.* April 30, 2018. https://healthitanalytics.com/news/top-12-ways-artificial-intelligence-will-impact-healthcare

Brown B. "Top 7 Health Care Trends and Challenges from Our Financial Expert." *Health Catalyst.* February 10, 2015. https://www.healthcatalyst.com/top-healthcare-trends-challenges

Esteva, A., A. Robicquet, B. Ramsundar, V. Kuleshov, M. DePristo, K. Chou, C. Cui, G. Corrado, S. Thrun, and J. Dean. "A Guide to Deep Learning in Health Care. *Nat Med* 25, no. 1 (2019): 24–29.

Frellick, M. "Will AI Make Physicians Obsolete?" *Medscape.* November 8, 2018. https://www.medscape.com/viewarticle/904626

Frellick, M. "AI Use in Health Care Increasing Slowly Worldwide." *Medscape.* May 6, 2019. https://www.medscape.com/viewarticle/912629

Frey, C.B., and M.A. Osborne. "The Future of Employment: How Susceptible Are Jobs to Computerisation?" *Technol Forecast Soc* 114 (2017): 254–280.

Frost & Sullivan. "Role of Blockchain in Precision Medicine." https://ww3.frost.com/files/3115/2050/6093/Edited_Frost_Prospective_-_Role_Of_Blockchain_in_Precision_Medicine_2nd_March_PS.pdf

Gawande, A. "Why Doctors Hate Their Computers." *The New Yorker.* November 28, 2018. https://www.newyorker.com/magazine/2018/11/12/why-doctors-hate-their-computers

Gershgorn, D. "If AI Is Going to Be the World's Doctor, It Needs Better Textbooks." *Quartz.* September 16, 2018. https://qz.com/1367177/if-ai-is-going-to-be-the-worlds-doctor-it-needs-better-textbooks/

Kaur, M. "Top 10 Real-Life Examples of Machine Learning." *Big Data Made.* May 13, 2019. https://bigdata-madesimple.com/top-10-real-life-examples-of-machine-learning/

Kayyali, B, D. Knott, and S.V. Kuiken. "The Big-Data Revolution in US Health Care: Accelerating Value and Innovation." *McKinsey and Co.* April 21, 2013. https://www.mckinsey.com/industries/healthcare-systems-and-services/our-insights/the-big-data-revolution-in-us-health-care

Kermany, D.S., M. Goldbaum, W. Cai, W., C.C. Valentim, H. Liang, S.L. Baxter, A. McKeown, G. Yang, X. Wu, F. Yan, and J. Dong. "Identifying Medical Diagnoses and Treatable Diseases by Image-based Deep Learning." *Cell* 172, no. 5 (2018): 1122–1131.

Lavery, T. "Quiz: Find Out How Smart You Are about Machine Learning and AI." *TechTarget.* June 29, 2020. https://searchenterpriseai.techtarget.com/quiz/Quiz-Find-out-how-smart-you-are-about-machine-learning-and-AI

LeCun, Y., Y. Bengio, and G. Hinton. "Deep Learning." *Nature* 521, no. 7553 (2015): 436–444.

Lin, S.Y., M.R. Mahoney, and C.A. Sinskey. "Ten Ways Artificial Intelligence Will Transform Primary Care." *J Gen Intern Med* 34, no. 8 (2019): 1–5.

"Machine Learning: What It Is and Why It Matters." *SAS.* https://www.sas.com/en_us/insights/analytics/machine-learning.html

Manyika, J. "A Future That Works: Automation, Employment, and Productivity." *McKinsey Global Institute.* January 2017. https://www.mckinsey.com/~/media/mckinsey/featured%20insights/Digital%20Disruption/Harnessing%20automation%20for%20a%20future%20that%20works/MGI-A-future-that-works-Executive-summary.ashx

Meskó, B., G. Hetényi, and Z. Győrffy. "Will Artificial Intelligence Solve the Human Resource Crisis in Health Care?" *BMC Health Serv Res* 18, no. 1 (2018): 545.

Pianin E. "US Health Care Costs Surge to 17 Percent of GDP." *The Fiscal Times.* December 3, 2015. http://www.thefiscaltimes.com/2015/12/03/Federal-Health-Care-Costs-Surge-17-Percent-GDP

Rajkomar, A., E. Oren, E, K. Chen, A.M. Dai, N. Hajaj, M. Hardt, P.J. Liu, X. Liu, J. Marcus, M. Sun, and P. Sundberg. "Scalable and Accurate Deep Learning with Electronic Health Records." *NPJ Dig Med* 1, no. 1 (2018): 18.

Russel, S., and P. Norvig. *Artificial Intelligence: A Modern Approach.* 3rd ed. Upper Saddle River, NJ: Pearson, 2010.

Zhao, R., R. Yan, Z. Chen, K. Mao, P. Wang, and R.X. Gao. "Deep Learning and Its Applications to Machine Health Monitoring." *Mech Syst Signal Pr* 115 (2019): 213–237.

References

1. McCarthy, J., M.L. Minsky, N. Rochester, and C.E. Shannon. "A Proposal for the Dartmouth Summer Research Project on Artificial Intelligence, August 31, 1955." *AI Mag* 27, no. 4 (2006): 12.
2. Szolovits, P., ed. *Artificial Intelligence in Medicine.* New York: Routledge, 2019.

3. Copeland, B.J. "Artificial Intelligence." *Encyclopedia Britannica*. https://www. britannica.com/technology/artificial-intelligence

4. Luxton, D.D. "Artificial Intelligence in Psychological Practice: Current and Future Applications and Implications." *Prof Psychol-Res Pr* 45, no. 5 (2014): 332–339.

5. Christensen, C.M. *The Innovator's Dilemma: When New Technologies Cause Great Firms to Fail*. Boston: Harvard Business Review Press, 2013.

6. Pearl, R. "Artificial Intelligence In Health Care: Separating Reality From Hype." *Forbes*. March 13, 2018. https://www.forbes.com/sites/robertpearl/2018/03/13/artificial-intelligence-in-healthcare/

7. Bouwens, J., and D.M. Krueger. "The Healthcare Industry Focuses On New Growth Drivers and Leadership Requirements." *Russell Reynolds Associates*. https://www.russellreynolds.com/insights/thought-leadership/embracing-change-the-healthcare-industry-focuses-on-new-growth-drivers-and-leadership-requirements

8. Silver, D., T. Hubert, J. Schrittwieser, and D. Hassabis. "AlphaZero: Shedding New Light on Chess, Shogi, and Go." Deep Mind [Blog post]. 2018. https://deepmind.com/blog/article/alphazero-shedding-new-light-grand-games-chess-shogi-and-go

9. Haenssle, H.A., C. Fink, R. Schneiderbauer, F. Toberer, T. Buhl, A. Blum, A. Kalloo, A.B.H. Hassen, L. Thomas, A. Enk, and L. Uhlmann. "Man Against Machine: Diagnostic Performance of a Deep Learning Convolutional Neural Network for Dermoscopic Melanoma Recognition in Comparison to 58 Dermatologists. *Ann Oncol* 29, no. 8 (2018): 1836–1842.

10. Bhardwaj, R., A.R. Nambiar, and D. Dutta, D. "A Study of Machine Learning in Health Care." *2017 IEEE 41st Annual Computer Software and Applications Conference (COMPSAC)* 2 (2017): 236–241. https://doi.org/10.1109/COMPSAC.2017.164

11. Olson, P. "This AI Just Beat Human Doctors on a Clinical Exam." Forbes. June 28, 2018. https://www.forbes.com/sites/parmyolson/2018/06/28/ai-doctors-exam-babylon-health/

12. Autor, D. "Polanyi's Paradox and the Shape of Employment Growth." Working Paper. Working Paper Series, National Bureau of Economic Research. September 2014. https://doi.org/10.3386/w20485

13. Bouwens, J., and D.M. Krueger. "Embracing Change: The Health Care Industry Focuses on New Growth Drivers and Leadership Requirements." *Russell Reynolds Associates*. https://www.russellreynolds.com/insights/thought-leadership/embracing-change-the-healthcare-industry-focuses-on-new-growth-drivers-and-leadership-requirements

14. "Tax Policy Center Briefing Book- Key Elements of the U.S. Tax System." *Tax Policy Center*. 2019. https://www.taxpolicycenter.org/sites/default/files/briefing-book/how_much_does_the_federal_government_spend_on_health_care.pdf

15. Rickert, J. "Patient-Centered Care: What It Means and How to Get There [Blog post]" *Health Affairs*. January 24, 2012. https://www.healthaffairs.org/do/10.1377/hblog20120124.016506/full/

16. Manyika, J. "A Future That Works: Automation, Employment, and Productivity." *McKinsey Global Institute*. January 2017. https://www.mckinsey.com/~/media/mckinsey/featured%20insights/Digital%20Disruption/Harnessing%20automation%20for%20a%20future%20that%20works/MGI-A-future-that-works-Executive-summary.ashx

17. Arntz, M., T. Gregory, and U. Zierahn. *The Risk of Automation for Jobs in OECD Countries*. Paris: OECD, 2016. https://doi.org/10.1787/5jlz9h56dvq7-en

18. Chui, M., J. Manyika, M., and Miremadi, "Where Machines Could Replace Humans—and Where They Can't (Yet)." *McKinsey Quarterly* 30, no. 2 (2016): 1–9.

19. Vardi, M.Y. "Artificial Intelligence: Past and Future." *Communications of the ACM* 55, no. 1 (2012): 5.

20. Vardi, M.Y. "Humans, Machines, and the Future of Work." *Plus Magazine*. https://plus.maths.org/content/humans-machines-and-future-work

21. Wartman, S.A., and C.D. Combs, "Reimagining Medical Education in the Age of AI." *AMA J Ethics* 21, no. 2 (2019): E146–E152. https://doi.org/10.1001/amajethics.2019.146

22. Raghupathi, W., and V. Raghupathi. "Big Data Analytics in Health Care: Promise and Potential." *Health Info Sci Syst* 2, no. 3 (2014): 1–10.

5
Professional Boundaries and Digital Professionalism

Physicians have a special relationship with their patients that is based on trust, which is a foundation for clinical care. Physicians have a fiduciary duty to care for their patients; that is, they put their patients' needs above their own. In return, patients put their unadulterated trust in the abilities and intentions of their doctors. However, there is another component that is crucial in protecting the interests of both the physician and the patient: professional boundaries. Professional boundaries are defined as often-unspoken, reciprocally understood limits that are placed within a professional relationship. These limits can be physical, emotional, sexual, or monetary in nature.

There are some professional boundaries that we become aware of early on in the process of professionalization that are inflexible and should never be crossed. However, many of the moral, ethical, and professional dilemmas that we encounter in the clinical setting are more nuanced. Furthermore, outside the confines of a healthcare institution, professional boundaries may not be as clearly established and should be adapted to the particular situation. For example, in end-of-life situations during home healthcare, emotional attachments to patients and family members may blur the lines of professional boundaries.[1] Additionally, the medical environment is rapidly changing due to advances in technology, and as a result, the boundaries of professionalism are constantly redefined. Digital professionalism—including communications via social media, information stored in healthcare systems, and use of mobile technology—continues to grow in importance.

Boundaries within the patient–physician relationship

Physicians regularly perform procedures that cross over the boundaries present in almost every other relationship. In the clinical setting, we often learn sensitive personal information, and conversations sometimes go beyond those necessary for purely medical purposes. But, how far is too far? What actions remain taboo in this unique relationship? There are specific ethical guidelines and laws provided by professional medical societies and also at the federal, state, and institutional levels that define professional boundaries. The same issue may have varied guidelines from different jurisdictions and organizations. For example, the concept of physicians writing prescriptions for themselves and their family members is interpreted and regulated very differently in different states and by different professional organizations. Therefore, it is recommended that physicians follow the most conservative guidelines.

Nearly all physicians enter the field of medicine with good intentions and practice with integrity. Only about 0.5 percent of physicians are the subject of state medical board disciplinary action each year, and only approximately 0.1 percent are the subject of severe actions involving revocation, suspension, or surrender of their license.[2] However, even physicians with good intentions are subject to lapses in professional conduct. The concept of the "slippery slope" can readily be applied to boundary concerns (see Figure 5.1). One step in the direction of impropriety can sometimes lead to further lapses, which may compound and eventually risk damaging personal and professional relationships or jeopardizing our medical licenses.

Treating family members or self-treatment

Treating a family member may complicate the physician–patient relationship and serve as a potential opportunity for boundary violations. The American Medical Association (AMA) generally recommends against physicians treating their immediate family members, because physicians may be hesitant to perform more sensitive aspects of a physical examination, or family members may be more wary to disclose sensitive medical information.[3] Informed consent becomes more difficult as well, as family members may not want to offend their relative by refusing his or her care or

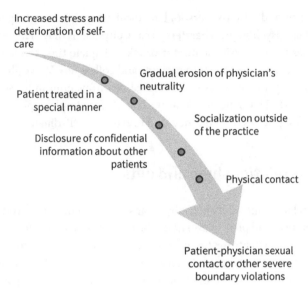

Increased stress and deterioration of self-care

Patient treated in a special manner

Gradual erosion of physician's neutrality

Disclosure of confidential information about other patients

Socialization outside of the practice

Physical contact

Patient-physician sexual contact or other severe boundary violations

Figure 5.1 The slippery slope.

recommendations. Physicians may also feel uncomfortable refusing to provide care for an inquiring relative. Children are at special risk, as they may be more likely to withhold sensitive information from a family member and less likely to be able to muster up the courage required to refuse care from a family member or their parents. The AMA concedes that family relations may be acceptable in routine care or in emergency situations, but treating family members can constitute a slippery slope and jeopardize both care and familiar relationships. Physicians should be particularly careful to document care provided to a family member. A lack of medical records can put the family member at risk physically and the physician at risk legally.

Similarly, physicians should be aware of the risks of treating themselves. Frequently referred to as the Father of Modern Medicine, Sir William Osler once said, "A physician who treats himself has a fool for a patient."[4] Physicians who treat themselves often keep incomplete records, have implicit bias in their self-examinations, and may attempt diagnoses and treatments outside their areas of expertise. Why, then, do some physicians choose to treat themselves? Just as patients may be reluctant to reveal personal information to family members who are physicians, physicians may be reluctant to sacrifice their privacy and discuss personal medical issues with colleagues. Even without these psychological barriers to care, physicians may believe that they cannot miss work to visit the doctor or take adequate time to recover from an illness due to commitment to patients and colleagues. We've all heard the lore of emergency room physicians requesting intravenous fluids so they can return to work. Nevertheless, treating oneself for simple conditions could constitute a slippery slope and may lead to errors in self-diagnosis.

Business relationships and gifts

Business relationships between physicians and patients may produce conflicts of interest, and physicians should be careful not to use information disclosed in medical visits for financial gain. Poor medical outcomes may also produce strain on business relationships, or vice versa. Physicians should carefully consider these factors before engaging in a physician–patient relationship with a friend or partner.

Gifts from patients may also affect the physician–patient relationship. The problem stems from perhaps a less-obvious tenet of professionalism: commitment to equitable provision of care. Gifts may have different meanings for the giver and receiver. Patients who give gifts typically do so with good intentions to express gratitude. Unfortunately, gift giving may lead to inadvertent favoritism or privilege, thus coloring further interactions. Special favors to patients—such as longer appointments, more attentive service, or other clinical advantages—could potentially lead down the slippery slope. Many institutions have clear guidelines that restrict the type of gifts that physicians are allowed to receive from patients. For example, the Mayo Clinic requires that all gifts of money and all gifts of substantial value that cannot be refused graciously must be forwarded to the Department of Development, which will handle the gift as a legal donation.

As a general guideline, the AMA Code of Medical Ethics, Opinion 1.2.8, suggests that physicians who receive gifts consider four things:

1. How does the gift compare to the patient's and physician's means? Gifts that are disproportionately large should be refused.
2. Will accepting the gift (or even being offered the gift) influence the patient's access to, or quality of, care?

3. Will the provision of the gift cause any emotional or financial hardship to the patient or their family?
4. Could it be more ethically appropriate to suggest a charitable donation in lieu of a gift? [5]

The AMA has one final recommendation for those who are still indecisive: consider whether you would be embarrassed to have colleagues find out that you had accepted the gift.

Sexual or romantic relationships

Forming a sexual or romantic relationship with a patient constitutes a special category of physician–patient violations and brings up ethical concerns due to the inherent power dynamics. Although the AMA says that physicians must at a minimum end the physician–patient relationship before beginning a sexual or romantic one, some state medical boards consider sexual or romantic relationships with former patients also to be instances of sexual misconduct.[6]

Additionally, some may also consider sexual relationships with *key third parties* to raise ethical issues. Key third parties include anyone who plays a significant role in the treatment of a patient, such as a spouse, parent, or guardian. The more involved this person is in decision-making for the patient, the more troubling a sexual or romantic relationship with the physician is. The AMA exhorts physicians to carefully consider whether they are compromising care or abusing their influence over the key third party before beginning such a relationship. Some state medical boards take a stricter stance and consider any romantic or sexual relationships with a key third party to be inappropriate. Governments at multiple levels also have established laws regarding the legality of and punishment for certain physician–patient relationship transgressions. Therefore, physicians must consider both ethical and legal guidelines before engaging in any sexual or romantic relationship with a former patient or key third party.

Despite the considerable policies about and punishments for patient sexual contact put forward by associations and boards, some physicians are still not dissuaded. In a nationwide survey of physicians, 4 percent of respondents reported that they had dated patients, 3 percent said they had had sex with a former patient, and 3 percent said they had had sex with a current patient.[7] In another survey, almost 7 percent of physicians self-reported a history of sexual relationships with patients.[8] Another survey indicated that 9 percent of physicians were not opposed to sexual contact between patient and physician.[9] Less than 1.6 percent of physicians are disciplined for sexual boundary violations with their patients, but according to self-reports, the incidence of sexual contact with patients is higher than those that are disciplined by as much as 330 percent.

Boundaries within the physician–trainee relationship

The supervisor–trainee relationship also requires special consideration within our profession. Based on the Association of American Medical College Graduation Questionnaire, data show that medical student mistreatment has been widespread for decades. Of the 2019 graduating medical school class, 40.4 percent of students expressed that they had personally suffered mistreatment.[10] Mistreatment in the form of public humiliation is likely a result of "pimping," a common practice in which supervisors will ask a trainee a series of difficult, sometimes unanswerable questions in quick succession.[11] Their answers, or lack thereof, are sometimes met with derogatory comments about the trainee's knowledge. Proponents of pimping suggest that it can encourage students to study harder, build camaraderie among the class, and act as practice for the high-pressure environments often found in the medical profession. Critics argue, however, that pimping can create a hostile learning environment, suppress creativity and curiosity, and result in students who feel harassed and dehumanized.[12]

Pimping doesn't present the only opportunity for medical student mistreatment. Students may be subject to sexual harassment or racist or sexist remarks. Occasionally, students may suffer from abuses of power by their superiors or have their evaluations used punitively. These actions are not only unethical but may also create a cycle of persistent unprofessionalism. Students may see successful, well-regarded physicians insulting their students, shoving trainees out of the way during procedures, or speaking in racially charged terms, and begin thinking that the fundamentals of professionalism are not needed to succeed in medicine. In this regard, the hidden curriculum serves to poison the well-intended lessons taught about professionalism in the formal curriculum.

When trainees who were treated poorly eventually come to have trainees of their own, they may feel entitled to treat them as poorly as they were treated, creating a vicious cycle of misconduct. There becomes a sense that abusive training is necessary to produce effective doctors. However, evidence shows that trainee abuse produces symptoms of posttraumatic stress and decreases career satisfaction in addition to decreasing confidence in the trainees' abilities.[13] Medical training is already difficult enough without the added emotional trauma of mistreatment. Virtually every student enters medical school with extraordinary study skills, a honed ability to comprehend, analyze, and apply voluminous information, and a service-driven mindset. Do we really to make the process more difficult for them?

Attempts to address medical school student mistreatment

The difficulty of minimizing student mistreatment in medical school is illustrated by a study undertaken at the David Geffen School of Medicine at the University of California at Los Angeles (DGSOM).[13] To address the problem of medical student mistreatment, DGSOM established the Gender and Power Abuse Committee in 1995. Third-year medical students were surveyed each year from 1996 to 2008 to assess the type, severity, and number of instances of mistreatment. Several additional measures were also instituted to reduce the number and severity of abuses, including the creation of an ombudsman office for the resolution of complaints, the establishment of a mechanism for formal reporting and investigation of incidents of abuse, and implementation of several comprehensive training programs. Although rates of reported abuse declined immediately after the committee released its "Statement on Supporting an Abuse-Free Academic Community," rates remained rather stable throughout the rest of the study. The additional training and resources failed to further decrease the reports of abuse. Additionally, the severity of reported mistreatments did not decline over the study period, and, in general, the percentage of students who sought to report and resolve instances of mistreatment did not increase during the period. Even after these multiyear interventions were implemented, the incidence of mistreatment at DGSOM was still near the national average at the end of the study.

So, what happened? The authors of the study concluded that their formal attempts at negating the hidden curriculum were not sufficient to prevent physicians and nurses from treating trainees the way they themselves had been treated. Medical professionals' perspectives on medical education and training have often been tainted by abuse they have experienced or observed, even if it is implicit. Furthermore, like every other medical school, DGSOM does not operate in a vacuum. Localized change may be hard to affect without systemic change throughout the profession.

What will it take to create long-lasting systemic change? The problem of violations in the physician–trainee relationship is a complex issue that may be better illuminated by also viewing them in the context of physician well-being. Steps to mitigate individual physician stressors by reviewing their causes and building upon physicians' coping strategies may be part of the solution (see Chapter 10 of this volume). Although no individual solution will be a panacea for eliminating mistreatment, exploring these other potential etiologies may be steps in the right direction.

Professional boundaries in the digital age

With the increased use of social media and other digital technologies, the struggle to maintain appropriate boundaries has taken on a whole new dimension. Social media and other forms of online interaction have increased ease of physician–patient interaction. As a result, the guidelines to proper conduct have been blurred, and the necessity of digital professionalism has been established. Is it okay to friend a patient on Facebook? Is it acceptable to search the internet for more information on a patient or to determine the veracity of what the patient has stated during an appointment? Can medical information be sent to patients via email? Can physicians text their patients or message them on Facebook or Twitter? While the internet provides physicians access to more information about their patients than ever before, it also provides additional considerations about the potential for violations of privacy. The understanding of digital professionalism will surely continue to develop as social media and other forms of technology become more widespread in the profession. However, it is still helpful to consider the potential for ethical violations before deciding to hit that "accept" button.

The first question physicians must consider when using social media is "Am I protecting patient privacy?" The Health Insurance Portability and Accountability Act of 1996 (HIPAA) was written to reform certain aspects of American healthcare, specifically health insurance. Perhaps its most well-known provision is Title II, which includes the HIPAA Privacy Rule that protects all identifying protected/personal health information (PHI) in every form, including paper, oral, and digital records. PHI includes information that is directly identifying—such as name, address, or date of birth—as well as any information that could be used to identify a patient, such as medical condition or services rendered. As with most regulations and laws, there is no leniency for physicians who do not know the guidelines. Even if done without awareness, sharing PHI and other protected information on social media is a violation of HIPAA. Patients' expectations of privacy demand that their stories remain their own and do not become yours to tell.[14]

Additional patient privacy concerns exist because of the popularity of posting photos and videos on the internet. Videos of procedures taken for educational purposes can expose the identity of the patient if certain identifying marks such as tattoos or other features are present. Taking photos of patients without their consent is ethically problematic and is strictly prohibited. The patient's needs ought to come before your own desire to share an interesting condition or thought-provoking experience. While some photos and videos taken in clinical settings may be shared in the best interest of public health and awareness, fully informed consent must be obtained, and every precaution should be taken to secure the patient's privacy.

Patient privacy isn't the only aspect that must be considered when a physician uses social media. There is also level of respect and professionalism expected from physicians at all times, including when they post on social media. Physicians may sometimes be drawn to social media to vent about difficult patients, frustrating cases, and healthcare mishaps. Even if patient privacy is protected in these cases, these kinds of posts reflect poorly on the physician and may lead to decreased trust for a patient. While venting to other physicians is an understandable practice when difficulties are inevitably encountered in the profession, venting online has the potential to reach an unintended audience and jeopardize the trust inherent in the physician–patient relationship. Text posts may be taken out of context or misconstrued, or patients may think that they are being referred to in a post when they are not. Even with privacy restrictions, social media is never quite as private as you think. Anything posted online has the potential to remain in circulation on the internet indefinitely.

The concept of digital professionalism may seem difficult to grasp at first. Let's look at a real-world example of when medical professionalism was undermined through the use of social media. A nursing student was dismissed from the University of Louisville after blogging about a childbirth she had attended.[15] Although much of what was written was not professional or proper (childbirth is "like being ripped apart by rabid monkeys;" "pregnancy makes an ok-looking woman ugly, and an ugly woman—f——— horrifying."), the expulsion was for reasons of patient privacy. The nursing student had written about specific medical procedures that she had witnessed, and even though the mother-to-be had consented to the nurse writing about her, it was only to allow the nurse to complete assignments associated with her training. The dismissed student brought a lawsuit against the University of Louisville because she felt that her First Amendment rights had been violated. However, the U.S. Court of Appeals for the Sixth Circuit ruled in favor of the university, saying that educational institutions could, in some instances, censor what students wrote online to uphold their missions. This was especially true because the student had signed an agreement at the beginning of her training agreeing to the privacy policies of the institution. More interestingly, perhaps, is that the Court of Appeals determined that the dismissal was for academic reasons, which require a significantly lower burden of proof, instead of conduct reasons. In essence, because the university was teaching medical professionalism, the student's online actions were an academic concern.[16]

Many students receive reprimands or punishment because of what they post online. In one survey, 60 percent of responding medical schools reported incidents of unprofessional online content (e.g., violation of patient privacy; use of profanity; depiction of intoxication; speaking about the medical profession in a negative tone), with 30 schools issuing informal warnings and three schools reporting instances of student dismissal.[17] Transgressions occurring as early as the first year of medical school may affect evaluations, job prospects, and the ability to continue to study medicine, so learners should seek to develop a professional identity around the principles of digital professionalism early on.

Is it appropriate to search for patients on the internet?

Consider the following case. A 35-year-old patient is in poor health, and you have advised him to cease smoking and drinking alcohol in excess, both of which have been components of his lifestyle for the past 15 years or so. You have presented him with numerous therapies, strategies, and resources for smoking cessation and have suggested ways in which he might still attend social events while avoiding the urge to drink too much. During one appointment, your patient reveals that all your conversations have paid off and that he has been living a much healthier lifestyle since his last appointment a month ago. You are suspicious of this sudden change of heart and prod for more details, but your patient is unwavering in his apparent commitment to good health. After he leaves, your suspicions lead you to an online search of your patient, and you quickly find his Facebook page complete with photos of him smoking cigarettes and a short video of him drinking liquor from the bottle, all dated within the past couple weeks. You resolve to continue counseling this patient to change his habits. But is obtaining information about patients online considered to be an appropriate thing for physicians to do?

Although a web search may turn up information pertinent to a patient's care, and this information may be publicly available on sites such as Facebook, Instagram, or Twitter, it is likely that this patient did not expect his physician to search for and obtain this information, constituting a perceived violation of privacy. Patients may lose their trust in their physician when they feel their privacy is being disregarded and may be more reticent in sharing important medical information with their physician. Furthermore, because information online may be prone to inaccuracies or falsehoods, basing medical decisions on evidence found on the internet may be harmful. For example, the photos and video of the patient may have been taken over a month ago and only recently posted. Photos of a patient could also potentially be biased due to the patient adopting an online persona.

Obtaining information about patients online may also complicate your decision-making process. Once you know (or think you know) about a patient's health habits because of what you saw on his or her online profile, you cannot "un-know" it, and it must influence your practice. If your current care plan is contraindicated by what you see online, you cannot, in good conscience, carry out your plan. You may have to confront your patient with the information for confirmation and decide on a new plan of action. However, if the patient denies the accuracy of what you saw online and insists that you carry on with his or her care as planned, you may be faced with an ethical dilemma. Establishing trust with the patient and obtaining clinical information directly are preferable to trying to find information online.

Finally, searching online may lead to poor quality of care even if health information is not found. What if you discover a patient's social media post excoriating your preferred political candidate? What if a Google search reveals a patient's criminal history? What if an Instagram photo shows a patient wearing a T-shirt that perpetuates a racial stereotype? Any number of things could come up from a quick online search, and there is no telling how they may affect your ability to provide unbiased care. It is usually preferable to operate only with information that the patient feels comfortable providing to you. Adding or looking up patients on social media may blur the boundaries of the physician–patient relationship and provide the physician with more information than they bargained for.

There are situations when an internet search of a patient may be justified. Emergency departments may use internet searches to obtain more information about patients for whom very little identifying information is available. Psychiatrists may be able to determine the accuracy of a patient's account quickly through a search, thus clarifying potential diagnoses and avoiding improper or unnecessary treatment. As online privacy policies continue to evolve alongside our understanding of medical professionalism on the internet, a more informed understanding of when an online search is merited may be continued to be shaped. Regardless, being aware of the risks associated with looking up a patient is important in deciding whether a patient's best interest is served when you look them up online.[18]

Communicating with patients online

Is it appropriate for physicians to communicate with patients using the internet? Many physicians now use email as a mode of communication with patients, and social media may soon follow. However, any identifying health information must be kept private. Some forms of online communication, although billed as "private," may be susceptible to hacks or leaks. It also may be impossible to confirm that the patient whose health information you are revealing is the one requesting and receiving the information online. Safeguards must be in place to make sure that patients' private information does not fall into the wrong hands. This is made more difficult by the fact that patients' health information may also be requested by insurers and consulting medical professionals. It is important that secure methods of storage and transfer of confidential health information are used. Many institutions have specific systems set up to provide for this security. It is a good idea to always use the methods approved by your institution; if there is no system in place, it is probably best to follow the traditional face-to-face method.

Once a physician begins engaging in online conversation with a patient, a bevy of new ethical considerations arise. For example, if you begin answering a patient's questions online, do you always need to be available to answer their questions? Will differences in response rates between patients be construed as bias? The Federation of State Medical Boards and the American College of Physicians recommend the establishment of guidelines for the type of issues appropriate for online discussion.[19] They also recommend that online communication be reserved only for those who will seek in-person follow-up, so that physicians can make sure they have provided appropriate advice online and that they have all the information they need for a well-thought-out course of treatment. It may also be wise to establish clear expectations for how often and how quickly you will be responding to patients' online requests for medical instruction; you do not want to put yourself on call 24/7 or risk damaging the physician–patient relationship because of unmet expectations.

Physicians' presence on social media

As previously discussed, social media should not be the place to vent about difficult patients, payment structures, law changes, or other professional frustrations. Prospective or current patients who view these posts may be uncomfortable with their venom, wonder what such a doctor might say about them behind their backs, or simply disagree with the ideas put forward; these feelings may lead them to seek medical care elsewhere. Furthermore, a patient may feel uncomfortable if their physician expresses a strong preference for views online that differ from their own. And because of the power dynamic inherent in the physician–patient relationship, the patient may not feel comfortable talking about their beliefs with their physician

Even innocuous online content can cause harm to a physician's practice.

Physicians are held to a high standard of professionalism, even outside the workplace, and posts that include references to alcohol consumption, heavy partying, or lewd humor may be viewed by both patients and hospitals as unbecoming of them. One study found that 14 percent of a sample of surgical residents had posted potentially unprofessional content on their Facebook profiles, and 12 percent had clearly unprofessional content.[20] This is not an issue that necessarily solves itself as physicians get older and develop professionally; another study found that 10 percent of practicing surgeons had potentially unprofessional content on their Facebook profiles, while 5 percent had clearly unprofessional content.[21] The Federation of State Medical Boards and the AMA both recommend separate professional and personal social media accounts, with strict privacy controls to prevent personal posts from being seen by those outside your circle of friends.[22] Professional accounts can allow for the dissemination of public health knowledge and the advancement of a physician's practice, while well-controlled personal accounts can provide safe places to engage in "normal" social media use.[23,24]

Maintenance of professional social media accounts is also important for those applying to medical school or residency. In a survey of 1,200 residency program directors, 16.3 percent said that they had reviewed internet resources to learn more about a residency application, and 38.1 percent of those had ranked the applicant lower as a result.[25] Program directors may view not only posts, but pictures, and *likes* or *favorites* of other people's content. By looking at social media, program directors or admissions committees may even find information that speaks favorably of an applicant's ability to survive and thrive in their program. Social media profiles may indicate that candidates are well-rounded and have good communication skills, a professional image, a pleasant personality that would fit well into their school or hospital, and whether they have a support structure of close family and friends.

The positive impacts of physicians utilizing social media

To this point, it may seem that social media only makes a physician's responsibilities more complex. The main concerns surrounding physicians' use of social media seem to center around maintaining a professional image, ensuring patient privacy and confidentiality, and being held accountable for the information that you share. Perceived time constraints and lack of experience have also been cited as barriers for adoption of the use of social media as a professional tool.[26] However, if these risks and barriers can be managed, social media can act as a great platform to network professionally, provide opportunities for collaboration, and share medical information with other physicians.[27] Social media has also been described as a tool for lifelong learning in today's information-sharing society.[28]

Social media can also be used to increase the visibility of our profession, and to share evidence-based medicine with the public. Dr. Bryan Vartabedian shared an example of this, in which he suggested that we, as physicians, have an ethical obligation to discuss health-related content online:

> Sound reasoning, good clinical information, and evidence-based thinking need to be part of the information stream. And doctors could change the way the world thinks if they would only get together to help create the information that patients see. Consider, for example, the issue of vaccines and autism. If you search for these subjects on Google, you will find the first two pages of search results contain anti-vaccine propaganda created by a loud, socially savvy minority. The American Academy of Pediatrics has 60,000 members. If every AAP member wrote a myth-dispelling blog post just once a year, Google would be ruled by reason. The medical community has the capacity and power to put good information where our patients seek it—we just need to make it a priority.[29p442]

While some physicians may be more comfortable sharing their work through peer-reviewed journals, microblogging has emerged as a way to share information rapidly and to a broader audience. Twitter has emerged as the main platform for medical professionals to discuss new research, crowd-source new ideas, and build communities of practice. Its character limit allows for information to be quickly processed. Many research journals now tweet information about articles and ask for contributors' Twitter handles at submission. Twitter use has also surged at medical conferences as a way for attendees to share information with the broader community.[30]

A study found that over 57 percent of physicians found social media to be beneficial, engaging, and a good way to obtain current, high-quality information, and 60 percent of respondents thought that social media improved their quality of patient care.[31] The presence and role of social media will continue to expand in the medical professions. We should strive to use it as a tool for increased engagement and life-long learning, keeping in mind the potential for privacy and boundary violations.

Telemedicine

Telemedicine is among the most exciting ways in which technology is being used in modern medicine as a force multiplier for medical training, communication, and collaboration. Defined as "the use of electronic information and communications technology to provide and support healthcare when distance separates the participants," telemedicine allows physicians to evaluate, diagnose, and treat patients at a distance.[32p16] Furthermore, telemedicine may also allow for enhanced communication between all members of the healthcare system, for example, through the facilitation of rapid specialist consultations. Telemedicine has a clear role in emergency situations and in remote environments in which access to healthcare is difficult and has potential for training and clinical care use in low-income and rural regions. As such, telemedicine has wide-ranging impacts on working toward healthcare equity.

Nonetheless, the use of telemedicine is more effective for certain types knowledge transfer than others. Telemedicine projects involving the communication of tacit knowledge—defined as knowledge that cannot be easily written down and "has a personal component that makes it difficult to communicate to others in an understandable form"—have more positive results than teleconsultation and distance-learning projects that involve primarily the transfer of explicit knowledge.[33p144] This may be because the complex knowledge discovery and creation process associated with the communication of tacit knowledge requires a rich communication media, while explicit knowledge may be more effectively communicated through other means, such as email or phone.

To the dismay of many, utilization rates of installed telemedicine projects have been consistently low, despite major advances in both capability and affordability of technology. Areas in which telehealth may be most effective, such as rural and underserved communities, may not have the proper infrastructure or resources to incorporate it. Concerns with privacy, safety, medical licensing, and reimbursement have prevented telemedicine from becoming widely adopted. For example, transmission of PHI through electronic means brings up additional concerns about patient privacy. Additionally, when state or international lines are crossed, it can be difficult to determine which laws apply. For example, must a physician in New York treating a patient in Kansas be licensed in both states? How does reimbursement work? There are many gray areas associated with the adoption of telemedicine, but legislations and regulations will have to evolve alongside the technology.

To minimize transmission risk, physicians and patients have turned to telemedicine during the COVID-19 pandemic. This has been a step toward widespread adoption, leading to temporary policy changes that have made telemedicine more accessible.[34] Direct-to-consumer telemedicine companies in particular have raised substantial investor capital and have been commercially successful. Telemedicine as a sector is a huge portion of the economy. Across 2018, investors poured a record-setting total of $8.1 billion into the sector, with 368 digital health deals with an average deal size of $21.9 million. The realm of direct-to-consumer products is dominated by a few major companies such as American Well and Teladoc, and companies such as Cerner and Epic have already built telehealth solutions into their platforms.

Electronic health records

The widespread adoption of electronic health records (EHRs) was spurred on by the promise of greater efficiency and improvements in care. Through market forces and the adoption of the Health Information Technology for Economic and Clinical Health Act in 2009, the proliferation of EHRs in the clinical environment has been dramatic: from 16 percent in 2008 to upwards of 90 percent today.[35] Governing and administrative bodies largely failed to take into account the physician experience in delivering care with EHRs, however, leading to alarming levels of physician dissatisfaction and burnout (see Chapter 10 of this volume). The widespread adoption of EHRs has also led to issues with patient privacy and safety. Of 1.735 million reported patient safety events in Pennsylvania from 2013 to 2016, 1,956 (0.11 percent) explicitly mentioned an EHR vendor or product and 557 (0.03 percent) explicitly suggested EHR usability contributed to possible patient harm.[36]

Not only do EHRs bring up novel concerns about the security and confidentiality of PHI, but they may also lead to issues with healthcare delivery. A new generation of physicians are experiencing patient encounters through the format of the EHR. As a result, they may not sufficiently develop the communication skills necessary for in-person treatment. Healthcare providers while inputting data during a patient encounter may miss psychological cues that are needed for communication, treatment, and compassionate care.[37] Furthermore, physicians who learned how to conduct patient encounters before the adoption of EHRs are struggling to adapt. The EHR system dictates an external framework for patient encounters, whereas physicians have already developed an internal framework of how to do this. As a result, many physicians have lost ownership of their own understanding of patients.

Chapter Quick Summary

- Professional boundaries are defined as often-unspoken, reciprocally understood limits that are placed within a professional relationship. These limits can be physical, emotional, sexual, or monetary in nature.
- Guidelines regarding the patient–physician relationship differ by institution, state, and professional organization, and physicians ought to understand all guidelines and follow the most conservative ones.
- Common opportunities for professional boundary violations with patients include treating family members, receiving gifts, and engaging in sexual or romantic relationships.
- The physician–trainee relationship has potential for boundary violations through mistreatment and "pimping."
- The widespread incorporation of digital technology and increased use of social media has led to further concerns about professional boundaries and patient privacy, establishing the necessity of digital professionalism.
- The adoption of telemedicine and EHRs may have benefits in streamlining healthcare delivery and improving access to healthcare, but there are considerable limitations in their current use today.

Resources

American Medical Association. "AMA Code of Medical Ethics Overview." July 9, 2019, https://www.ama-assn.org/delivering-care/ethics/code-medical-ethics-overview

American Medical Association. "AMA Digital Health Implementation Playbook." 2020. https://www.ama-assn.org/amaone/ama-digital-health-implementation-playbook

Hasty, B.N., E. Brandford, and J.N. Lau. "It's Time to Address Student Maltreatment." *Rise (Research in Surgical Education)*, online journal, American College of Surgeons. Posted July 2018. Accessed at: https://www.facs.org/education/division-of-education/publications/rise/articles/student-mistreatment

References

1. Abrams, R., T. Vandrevala, K. Samsi, and J. Manthorpe. "The Need for Flexibility When Negotiating Professional Boundaries in the Context of Home Care, Dementia and End of Life." *Ageing Soc* 39, no. 9 (2019): 1976–1995, https://doi.org/10.1017/S0144686X18000375

2. DuBois, J.M., E.E. Anderson, J.T. Chibnall, J. Mozersky, and H.A. Walsh. "Serious Ethical Violations in Medicine: A Statistical and Ethical Analysis of 280 Cases in the United States from 2008–2016." *Am J Bioethics* 19, no. 1 (2019): 16–34. https://doi.org/10.1080/15265161.2018.1544305

3. American Medical Association. "AMA Code of Medical Ethics, Opinion 1.2.1." 2016. https://www.ama-assn.org/delivering-care/ethics/treating-self-or-family

4. Osler, W.S., and R.B. Bean. *Sir William Osler Aphorisms: From His Bedside Teachings and Writings.* Springfield, IL: C.C. Thomas, 1961.

5. American Medical Association. "AMA Code of Medical Ethics, Opinion 1.2.8." 2016. https://www.ama-assn.org/delivering-care/ethics/gifts-patients

6. American Medical Association. "AMA Code of Medical Ethics, Opinion 9.1.1." 2016. https://www.ama-assn.org/delivering-care/ethics/romantic-or-sexual-relationships-patients

7. Bayer, T., J. Coverdale, and E. Chiang. "A National Survey of Physicians' Behaviors Regarding Sexual Contact with Patients." *South Med J* 89, no. 10 (1996): 977–982.

8. Sansone R.A., and L.A. Sansone. "Crossing the Line: Sexual Boundary Violations by Physicians." *Psychiatry (Edgmont)* 6, no. 6 (June 2009): 45–48.

9. Regan, S., T.G. Ferris, and E.G. Campbell. "Physician Attitudes toward Personal Relationships with Patients." *Med Care* 48, no. 6 (2010): 547–552.

10. Association of American Medical Colleges. "Medical School Graduation Questionnaire 2019 All Schools Summary Report." August 2019. https://www.aamc.org/system/files/2019-08/2019-gq-all-schools-summary-report.pdf

11. Markman, J.D., T.M. Soeprono, H.L. Combs, and E.M. Cosgrove, "Medical Student Mistreatment: Understanding 'Public Humiliation." *Med Educ Online* 24, no. 1 (2019): 1615367. https://doi.org/10.1080/10872981.2019.1615367

12. McCarthy, C.P., and J.W. McEvoy, "Pimping in Medical Education: Lacking Evidence and Under Threat." *JAMA* 314, no. 22 (2015): 2347–2348. https://doi.org/10.1001/jama.2015.13570

13. Fried, J.M., M. Vermillion, N.H. Parker, and S. Uijtdehaage. "Eradicating Medical Student Mistreatment: A Longitudinal Study of One Institution's Efforts." *Acad Med* 87, no. 9 (2012): 1191–1198. https://doi.org/10.1097/ACM.0b013e3182625408

14. U.S. Department of Health and Human Services. "Summary of the HIPAA Privacy Rule." 2003. https://www.hhs.gov/hipaa/for-professionals/privacy/laws-regulations/index.html

15. Jaschik, S. "Appeals Court Upholds Blogging-related Expulsion of Student from Nursing School." *Inside Higher Education News.* June 6, 2013. https://www.insidehighered.com/news/2013/06/06/appeals-court-upholds-blogging-related-expulsion-student-nursing-school

16. Nina Yoder v. University of Louisville, 12-5354 (6th Cir. 2013).

17. Chretien, K.C., S.R. Greysen, J.-P. Chretien, and T. Kind. "Online Posting of Unprofessional Content by Medical Students." *JAMA* 302, no. 12 (2009): 1309–1315. https://doi.org/10.1001/jama.2009.1387

18. Genes, N., and J. Appel. "The Ethics of Physicians' Web Searches for Patients' Information." *J Clin Ethic* 26 (2015): 68–72.

19. Federation of State Medical Boards. "Social Media and Electronic Communications." 2019. http://www.fsmb.org/siteassets/advocacy/policies/social-media-and-electronic-communications.pdf

20. Langenfeld, S.J., G. Cook, C. Sudbeck, T. Luers, and P.J. Schenarts. "An Assessment of Unprofessional Behavior among Surgical Residents on Facebook: A Warning of the Dangers of Social Media." *J Surg Educ* 71, no. 6 (2014): e28–e32. https://doi.org/10.1016/j.jsurg.2014.05.013

21. Langenfeld, S.J., C. Sudbeck, T. Luers, P. Adamson, G. Cook, and P.J. Schenarts. "The Glass Houses of Attending Surgeons: An Assessment of Unprofessional

Behavior on Facebook Among Practicing Surgeons." *J Surg Educ* 72, no. 6 (2015): e280–e285. https://doi.org/10.1016/j.jsurg.2015.07.007

22. Sullivan, T. "Federation of State Medical Boards Model Policy Guidelines for Social Media." *Policy & Medicine*. May 6, 2018. https://www.policymed.com/2012/06/federation-of-state-medical-boards-model-policy-guidelines-for-social-media.html

23. Farnan, J.M., L.S. Sulmasy, B.K. Worster, H.J. Chaudhry, J.A. Rhyna, and V.M. Arora. "Online Medical Professionalism: Patient and Public Relationships: Policy Statement From the American College of Physicians and the Federation of State Medical Boards." *Ann Intern Med* 158, no. 8 (2013): 620. https://doi.org/10.7326/0003-4819-158-8-201304160-00100

24. American Medical Association. "Code of Medical Ethics, Opinion 2.3.2." 2016. https://www.ama-assn.org/delivering-care/ethics/professionalism-use-social-media

25. Go, P.H., Z. Klaassen, and R.S. Chamberlain. "Attitudes and Practices of Surgery Residency Program Directors Toward the Use of Social Networking Profiles to Select Residency Candidates: A Nationwide Survey Analysis." *J Surg Educ* 69 (2012): 292–300.

26. Antheunis, M.L., K. Tates, and T.E. Nieboer. "Patients' and Health Professionals' Use of Social Media in Health Care: Motives, Barriers and Expectations." *Patient Educ Couns* 92, no. 3 (2013): 426–431. https://doi.org/10.1016/j.pec.2013.06.020

27. Cheston, C.C., T.E. Flickinger, and M.S. Chisolm. "Social Media Use in Medical Education: A Systematic Review." *Acad Med* 88, no. 6, (2013): 893–901. https://doi.org/10.1097/ACM.0b013e31828ffc23

28. Kind, T., and Y. Evans. "Social Media for Lifelong Learning." *Int Rev Psychiatr* 27, no. 2 (2015): 124–132. https://doi.org/10.3109/09540261.2014.990421

29. Vartabedian, B.S. "Anonymous Physician Blogging: Commentary 1." *AMA J Ethic* 13, no. 7 (2011): 440–443. https://doi.org/10.1001/virtualmentor.2011.13.7.ccas3-1107

30. Paton, C., P.D. Bamidis, G. Eysenbach, M. Hansen, and M. Cabrer. "Experience in the Use of Social Media in Medical and Health Education." *Yearb Med Inform* 20, no. 1 (2011); 21–29. https://doi.org/10.1055/s-0038-1638732

31. McGowan, B.S., M. Wasko, B.S. Vartabedian, R.S. Miller, D.D. Freiherr, and M. Abdolrasulnia. "Understanding the Factors That Influence the Adoption and Meaningful Use of Social Media by Physicians to Share Medical Information." *J Med Internet Res* 14, no. 5 (2012): e117. https://doi.org/10.2196/jmir.2138

32. Field, M.J. "Introduction and Background." In *Telemedicine: A Guide to Assessing Telecommunications in Health Care*. Edited by M.J. Field. Washington, DC: National Academies Press, 1996.

33. Paul, D.L. "Collaborative Activities in Virtual Settings: A Knowledge Management Perspective of Telemedicine." *J Manage Inform Syst* 22, no. 4 (2006): 143–176. https://doi.org/10.2753/MIS0742-1222220406

34. Bashshur, R., C.R. Doarn, J.M. Frenk, J. C. Kvedar, and J.O. Woolliscroft. "Telemedicine and the COVID-19 Pandemic, Lessons for the Future." *Telemed E-Health* 26, no. 5 (2020): 571–573. https://doi.org/10.1089/tmj.2020.29040.rb

35. Office of the National Coordinator for Health Information Technology. "Office-Based Physician Electronic Health Record Adoption." *Health IT Dashboard*. 2017. https://dashboard.healthit.gov/quickstats/pages/physician-ehr-adoption-trends.php

36. Howe, J.L., K.T. Adams, A.Z. Hettinger, and R.M. Ratwani. "Electronic Health Record Usability Issues and Potential Contribution to Patient Harm." *JAMA* 319, no. 12 (2018): 1276–1278. https://doi.org/10.1001/jama.2018.1171

37. Sulmasy, L., A.M. Lopez, and C. Horwitch. "Ethical Implications of the Electronic Health Record: In the Service of the Patient." *J Gen Intern Med* 32, no. 8 (2017): 935–939. https://doi.org/10.1007/s11606-017-4030-1

6

Communication, Empathy, and Compassion

On average, physicians will conduct hundreds of thousands of medical evaluations and follow-ups throughout their career. In the past, communication skills were mostly learned through mentor–mentee relationships and clinical observations. However, given the incredible volume of communicative demand, medical schools and residency programs have recognized the need for effective communication and have increasingly moved toward integrating formal communication training into their curricula. Furthermore, many medical schools have embraced the holistic review process, incorporating effective communication skills and empathy as criteria for selecting candidates.[1]

In today's fast-paced medical environment, in which physicians feel pressure to see more patients in a limited amount of time, clinical interpersonal skills are more important than ever. Furthermore, we must consider the changing role of the physician as technological advances continue to transform the field of medicine. Artificial intelligence may soon outperform physicians in the diagnostic decision-making processes (see Chapter 4 of this volume). How do we position ourselves as physicians and adapt to these changes? What will remain constant is our role to communicate and engage with patients: "Medicine is an art whose magic and creative ability have long been recognized as residing in the interpersonal aspects of the patient-physician relationship."[2p18]

Effective communication benefits both patients and physicians

Research has shown that better health measured physiologically (blood pressure or blood sugar), behaviorally (functional status), or subjectively (patient self-evaluation of overall health status) can be consistently related to specific aspects of physician–patient interactions.[3] Effective physician–patient communication has also been shown to help regulate patients' emotions, improve comprehension of medical information and options, and allow for better identification of patients' specific needs, perceptions, and expectations.[4] In addition, patients are more likely to share information pertinent to their diagnoses, follow physician advice, and report satisfaction with their care. Patients' agreement with their doctor about the nature of their treatment and need for follow-up is strongly associated with positive recovery results.

If better treatment outcomes aren't incentive enough, physicians should also consider the changing landscape of physician evaluation and reimbursement. More than 75 percent of hospitals are now factoring patient satisfaction into their reimbursement calculations, and Medicare calculates patient satisfaction scores when determining payments under the Affordable Care Act.[5] Patients are often asked to score their physicians on metrics such as "Doctor spoke in clear language"; "Doctor showed concern for questions and worries"; and "Doctor explained the condition/problem well." While the concept of patient satisfaction seems logical and productive, it can also have unintended negative consequences. Seventy-eight percent of clinicians in one study said patient satisfaction scores moderately or severely affected their job satisfaction negatively, and 28 percent said the scores made them consider quitting.[6] However, there is potentially good news: research has shown that physician communication training may improve patient satisfaction scores.[7]

The majority of patients now consult online reviews when choosing a physician. Yelp, Healthgrades, Zocdoc, and other aggregators provide referrals as well as a platform for patients to voice their opinions about individual practitioners, private practices, and hospitals. Although patient reviews are questionable representations of a physician's clinical ability, they do provide valuable information for both patients and providers. A recent survey showed that over 65 percent of respondents were aware of physician-rating websites, and 35 percent had sought online physician reviews within the past year.[8] According to the same survey, among those who sought physicians' ratings online, 35 percent reported selecting a physician based on good ratings, and 37 percent reported avoiding a physician with bad ratings.

Counterintuitively, negative online ratings of physicians by patients mostly focus on poor communication and not about patient outcomes. As an example, in Zagat's Health Survey Tool, rated criteria include trust, communication, availability, and environment. None of the criteria explicitly ask patients to rate the technical expertise of the physician. A 2016 study showed no correlation between cardiac surgeons' average online rating and risk-adjusted mortality rates.[9] Although there are other factors influencing patient reviews of physicians including logistical issues in the office, waiting times, and infrastructure, communication is at the core of most ratings. According to the American Hospital Association,

> today's healthcare environment makes good communication among patients, families, and caregivers harder and harder to achieve. Hospital stays are shorter, medical care is more technologically complex, resources are constrained, and there is a growing need for patients and families to have more information about, and involvement in, care decisions.[10p1]

Research shows that physicians consistently overestimate their abilities in communication. For example, a study showed that 75 percent of orthopedic surgeons surveyed believed that they had satisfactory communication with patients, yet only 21 percent of their patients agreed.[11] Breakdown of communication can have disastrous consequences. Research has shown that communication was a factor in 30 percent of medical malpractice cases filed from 2009 to 2013.[12] In a recent systematic review of patient safety incidents in primary care, between 6 and 67 percent of incidents were found to be a result of administrative or communicative issues.[13] Furthermore, there are an estimated 1.2 million preventable adverse drug events each year due to errors in administering medication, much of which stems from issues in communication.[14] Additionally, 50 percent of patients over the age of 65 had medication discrepancies at hospital discharge and associated readmission and complication related to poor communication.[15] An estimated 80 percent of serious medical errors are attributed to mistakes in communication when responsibility for patients is transferred or handed off.[16] (We will discuss the concept of working as a healthcare team and the communication that needs to exist between members further in Chapter 8 of this volume.)

Effective communication is a requirement for patient-centered care

Three main purposes of physician–patient communication are creating a good interpersonal relationship, exchanging information, and making treatment-related decisions.[17] While researchers have wide-ranging definitions, some see the physician–patient relationship as one that is mostly social, citing elements such as laughing or making jokes, making personal remarks, giving patient compliments, conveying interest, general friendliness, honesty, a desire to help, devotion, and a nonjudgmental attitude and social orientation. Others see the main importance of the physician–patient relationship as therapeutic, a way to create mutual trust. These researchers subscribe to a patient-centered theory that has its roots in Carl Rogers's "client-centered" theory. In this theory, the information asymmetry between doctor and patient is flattened rather than highlighted, and the two parties are seen as equal. The patient leads in domains in which they have expertise, notably their symptoms, preferences, and expectations, while the physician leads in their domains of diagnosis and treatment, which creates an environment that enables frank and open discussion. The principles of patient-centered medicine date back to the ancient Greek school of Cos established by Hippocrates.

Until recently, paternalism, or physician-centered decision-making, reigned as the dominant model for delivery of medical care. For example, physicians considered it inhumane and detrimental to patients to disclose bad news, particularly about terminal cancer diagnoses. Since then, there has been a move from information transfer to information exchange and incorporating patients in decision-making as part of the clinical team.

Without a historical focus on formal curricula for developing communication skills in medicine, physicians largely may be left unprepared for the emotional intensity and communicative complexity of delivering bad news.[18] Physicians may feel that they will be blamed during the process or not know all of the answers, which may lead to emotional disengagement with patients.[19] However, a patient-centered approach in which physicians convey information according to the patient's needs has been shown to yield the most positive outcomes for patients on a cognitive, evaluative, and emotional level.[20] By sharing relevant information with patients, and subsequently checking for understanding and showing empathy, physicians are able to more effectively deliver bad news.

In a study conducted at the Baylor University Medical Center, 93 percent of the surgeons surveyed stated that delivering bad news was a very important skill, and 7 percent, a somewhat important skill.[21] However, only 43 percent of those surveyed felt that they had received adequate training in this important communication skill, highlighting the need for formal measures of communication training.

Many protocols for delivering bad news have been established in the literature, including the six-step SPIKES[22] protocol and the ABCDE model.[23] These protocols are similar, so we will only describe the SPIKES model. SPIKES stands for

S: *Setting up the interview*: Focusing on maximizing privacy, involving family members, maintaining eye contact, and removing barriers and interruptions from the physical environment.

P: *Assessing the patient's perception.* Asking the patient open-ended questions regarding their current understanding of specific information concerning their illness and diagnosis.

I: *Obtaining the patient's invitation.* Allowing the patient to direct the timing of the physician's disclosure of the bad news regarding tests, illness, or progress.

K: *Giving knowledge and information to the patient.* Information is best delivered by first warning the patient that bad news is coming and keeping the conversation at the level of comprehension of the patient.

E: *Addressing the patients emotions with empathic responses.* Patients may respond with varying emotional reactions including grief, sadness, shock, and anger. Empathic responses by the physician include observing the patient's emotions, guiding the patient to express their feelings and thoughts, and using verbal and nonverbal validating responses to express support.

S: *Strategy and summary*: Asking patients if they are ready for a discussion is crucial after delivering bad news. Revisit Step 2 (patient's perception) and repeatedly review the patient's unrealistic expectations, and then summarize the discussion in order to provide clarification and outline next steps.

Of course, the broad outline of patient-centered theory—or shared decision making, as it is sometimes referred to—leaves many details to be decided. For one, the question of how much information should be conveyed to patients has been complicated in recent years by the increasing use of big data models in medicine. These technologies allow for increasingly greater precision in the ability to predict risk for disease and treatment outcomes. The ability to estimate with increasing accuracy how long a patient might live without severe health complications raises important ethical questions about what information patients need to know to make informed healthcare decisions. For example, if an artificial intelligence model is able to predict how likely patients will die within a certain time period after finding out they have cancer, is it the responsibility of the physician to let them know? Physicians ought to keep in mind the clinically significant influences of hope, which, for example, has been shown to be associated with positive after-effects following invasive heart surgery and increased quality of life for patients in clinical trials for metastatic renal cell carcinoma.

Another ethically ambiguous aspect of shared decision-making is the way in which physicians ought to balance their clinical opinion with the wishes of the patient. A recent study considered the case of a neonatologist who was faced with the task of communicating with the parents of an infant with severe neurocognitive impairment and a bleak recovery prognosis. The physician was faced with telling the parents that they must decide between providing artificial respiration or end-of-life care to their child.[24] While physicians may feel that their medical expertise and experience with similar cases justify a more heavy-handed approach where they explicitly recommend a course of action, the authors of the study questioned this approach based on the shared decision-making model. The parents are, after all, ultimately responsibility emotionally and physically for the child long-term. This case shows just how nuanced and patient-specific communication demands can be for the physician.

Components of effective communication in medicine

There are many components of effective communication, including clear speech, management of tone, and empathy and respect. Three components that are particularly important for medical professionals are active listening, giving and receiving feedback, and the apology.

Active listening

In the words of Sir William Osler, "Listen to the patient, he is telling you the diagnosis."[25] Listening is an often-overlooked aspect of effective communication in the clinic. In a patient-centered approach, physicians allow patients to share their agendas, symptoms, and expectations. However, a study showed that patient agendas were only elicited in 36 percent of encounters, and that physicians, on average, interrupted patients within 11 seconds.[26] Ideally, physicians ought to adopt an *active* or *empathic* listening strategy.

Active listening was first discussed by Carl Rogers in 1951 as a cornerstone of humanistic psychology. It has emerged as a tool for effective communication in the clinical environment. Although the components of active listening differ from source to source, most proponents state that it has three parts: communicating nonverbal engagement and giving the speaker unconditional attention; paraphrasing the speaker's words and restating them to convey understanding; and asking questions to gain more information. It is important to note that active listening is both verbal and nonverbal. An often-cited statistic is that only 7 percent of communication is verbal, whereas 38 percent occurs through tone of voice, and 55 percent is nonverbal. Therefore, reading nonverbal cues such as facial expressions allows physicians to better understand patient's motivation and feelings.

Giving and receiving feedback

To be successful as medical students or professionals, we have consistently performed at the highest level in our studies. Furthermore, our profession requires us to minimize errors to ensure patient safety. Therefore, it is unsurprising that many of us expect perfection from ourselves professionally. However, professionalization is an ongoing process of learning and developing and requires first that we embrace the reality that we have room for improvement. Just as the reflective process is a vital tool for professional identity formation, feedback can help us to identify our strengths and weaknesses to grow professionally.

However, feedback may be difficult to give and receive. Learners may feel intimidated to ask for feedback because they feel that less-than-stellar feedback is a negative judgement of their ability. On the other hand, those giving feedback may be wary of how learners will react and not provide pertinent, growth-promoting information. Learning to both ask for and give effective feedback are important communication skills to develop as medical professionals.

There are two types of feedback: formative and summative. Formative feedback provides information about how learners can improve their knowledge and skills, while summative feedback refers to evaluation at the end of an event. While there is a need for summative feedback at times, formative feedback is nonevaluative and plays a greater role in supporting the goal-oriented process of improvement that is central to the concept of lifelong learning. The components of formative feedback are described in Box 6.1.

Box 6.1 The Components of Formative Feedback

Formative feedback is
- *Supportive*: provides reassurance about competency, can reduce uncertainty about whether a student is performing well or poorly on a task.
- *Timely*: offered close to the observed behavior before the learner or observer forgets.
- *Credible*: comes from a source who has observed the learner and who is knowledgeable about the material she or he is teaching.
- *Specific*: describes the observed behavior; verifies actions and elaborates.
- *Goal-directed*: identifies areas for improvement and comes up with a plan.
- *Objective*: compares learner to standards, although not with other students directly.
- *Joint effort*: requires assessment by both learner and teacher.

Source: A. Mariani, S. Schumann, H.B. Fromme, M. Zegarek, S. Swearingen, M. Ryan, and S. Reddy, "Asking for Feedback: Helping Learners Get the Feedback They Deserve," *MedEdPORTAL* 11 (2015), https://doi.org/10.15766/mep_2374-8265.10228.

The apology

Physicians have been leery of apologizing to patients because an apology could be viewed as a clear admission of guilt in a court of law. While physicians ought to be cautious about legal liability and should learn the laws of the state they practice in, evidence shows that showing concern for patients and communicating effectively when a medical error has been made can produce numerous benefits. These benefits include patient satisfaction, increased closure for both patient and physician, and reduced risk of liability for the physician. The Michigan model, developed by the University of Michigan Medical School in 2004, has been a seminal model for communicating with patients about medical errors; it can be summarized as follows: Apologize when appropriate while reflecting on the causes, explain and create a solid plan to defend when you are right, and commit to legal remedies only if all else fails.[27] The Michigan model showed that for physicians who disclosed medical errors, malpractice claims dropped 36 percent and lawsuits dropped 65 percent. Apology laws, which facilitate apologies by making them inadmissible as evidence in court, have been adopted in some form by the majority of state governments. The American Medical Association states in the Code of Medical Ethics that when a medical error has been made, physicians should

> disclose the occurrence of the error, explain the nature of the (potential) harm, and provide the information needed to enable the patient to make informed decisions about future medical care, as well as acknowledge the error and express professional and compassionate concern toward patients who have been harmed in the context of health care.[28]

Furthermore, the American Medical Association emphasizes that "concern regarding legal liability should not affect the physician's honesty with the patient."

How should a physician apologize? We suggest four distinct steps: acknowledgment, explanation, expression of remorse, and reparation (see Figure 6.1).

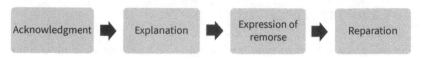

Figure 6.1 Components of an apology.

"Difficult" patients

The decision to become a medical professional often stems from an altruistic calling to care for others. It has never been enough to have a brilliant scientific mind or the tenacity to power through seemingly endless medical training. Healthcare providers have an incredibly difficult job, and a desire to work with patients through their problems is essential for physicians to find meaning in their work. Anecdotes abound of those who say that seeing patients is the absolute best part of their day. And yet, even these extremely dedicated individuals will struggle with patients they label as "difficult."

Up to 15 percent of patient encounters are labeled as "difficult" by the physicians providing care.[29] Physicians may label patients as "difficult" due to clinical challenges in treating their conditions or as a result of negative patient emotions, dispositions, or mental illnesses. Some "difficult" patients may be angry, extremely fearful of a diagnosis or treatment, or may be struggling with personality disorders.[30] Others may present with nonspecific symptoms that have been worked up to no avail. Many "difficult" patients may suffer from mental illnesses, making it challenging to appropriately provide treatment.[31] Patients with schizophrenia, bipolar disorder, or a personality disorder may have no physical illness at all, or their mental symptoms may obscure underlying physical symptoms. Furthermore, current trends in healthcare that limit physician time with patients and increase clerical burden are likely to be contributing to this "difficult" patient problem. Physicians who are unable to appropriately spend time engaging with patients and addressing the root of their problem may feel worn down and label these patients as "difficult."

Physicians who begin to feel worn down by "difficult" patients may, inadvertently, create a cycle of problematic encounters. Even when patients are perfectly affable and have no difficulty relating symptoms, the physician's emotions and opinions can weigh on the appointment. Often, anger held over from previous appointments can be misdirected at new patients. As an example, impatience bred from overlong dialogues with patients may cause a physician to have a clipped tone and a rushed manner through the next few patient encounters. Physicians who feel bitter about their lack of progress with one patient are apt to pay less attention to the medical problems of others. This can create more and more seemingly "difficult" patients until the physician feels overwhelmed and begins to grow cynical and disillusioned. When the joy of patient care is decreased, physicians may grow more cynical about their work. Allowing physicians the resources to appropriately engage with their patients is likely a part of the solution to dealing with "difficult" patients.

Digital communication

In today's medical environment, technology plays an increasing role. Communication through the digital space allows for timely and convenient responses. Patients increasingly desire communication through digital means, so physicians should develop digital communication skills. Digital communication encompasses two-sided communication with patients through email, instant messaging, online patient portals, and telemedicine. It also encompasses one-sided communication through maintaining an online reputation by creating accessible websites for your practice and connecting with the general public through social media and microblogging. (These kinds of persona-building communication activities are discussed further in the context of guidelines and boundaries for digital professionalism in Chapter 4 of this volume.) Whether we like it or not, healthcare is moving to providing services through the digital space. A report from the McKinsey Global Institute asserts that we can expect the majority of medical services to be digital in a few years.[32] Whether this comes to pass, some amount of communication and marketing and practice management will be in the digital space, whether it's Doximity or a physician-directed and Health Insurance Portability and Accountability Act–compliant software.[33]

Many of us are used to "Googling" ourselves regularly to see if there are any potentially negative comments online that could affect our businesses and reputation. Multiple ways to continuously monitor this in the form of online reputation management companies exist, which continuously scrub the internet and get rid of potential problematic comments.

The widespread incorporation of technology into medicine has worked to create a divide between the older and younger generations of physicians. The new generation grew up with an extra-normative component of how they relate to the world: technology. As a result, they are able to easily use technology as a tool for communication. On the other hand, the older generation has struggled more with the use of technology. Just as a person who learns a language later in their life will not truly incorporate it as a native speaker would, even as the older generation learns how to incorporate technology into their communication toolbox, they may not display the automatic proficiency of the younger generation.

Empathy

Empathy is a core feature of all types of shared decision-making. Patients often regard their doctors as one of their most important sources of psychological support. Therefore, empathy—often defined generally as the ability to understand and share the feelings of others—is a critical skill that physicians must possess. The desire to help and the ability to convey an understanding of the patient's situation are the most powerful ways of providing support to them. Furthermore, multiple studies have linked empathy with increased patient satisfaction, interpersonal trust between patients and physicians, compliance with physicians' recommendations, decreased patient anxiety and distress, better clinical outcomes, decreased physician burnout, and lower risk of malpractice suits.[34]

The nature of empathy has been debated by philosophers and psychologists for thousands of years. One particularly interesting perspective comes from author Leslie Jamison. She developed an understanding of empathy in medicine during her time working as a medical actor for doctors-in-training. In her book of essays, *The Empathy Exams*, she explains:

> Empathy comes from the Greek *empatheia*—em ("into") and pathos ("feeling")—a penetration, a kind of travel. It suggests you enter another person's feelings as you'd enter another country, border-crossing by way of query: What grows where you are? What are the laws? What animals graze here?[35p24]

Within the broad concept of empathy, there are many divisions. Morse's model for clinical empathy, which views empathy as a form of professional interaction, includes four components: emotive, moral, cognitive, and behavioral (see Table 6.1).[36]

Emotive empathy is what many people think about when they hear the word "empathy." Also referred to as affective empathy, emotive empathy describes the ability to subjectively experience another person's emotions and is largely an automatic process that is ingrained early on in life. In subjects with psychopathic tendencies, empathy dysfunction may be confined to affective empathy, because they do not possess the ability to feel the suffering of others.[37] Furthermore, physicians who engage too much in affective empathy may be prone to a response of empathic distress, which has been implicated in physician disengagement and burnout.

Moral empathy refers to an internal altruistic force that motivates empathy. *Cognitive empathy* is described as the ability to understand another's state of mind from an objective viewpoint and is also commonly referred to as perspective-taking. According to Halpern, the ability for objective emotional reasoning is the key for exercising clinical empathy.[38] Crucially, according to Morse, empathy is not only an emotional and cognitive process but is also actionable. *Behavioral empathy* refers to the communicative

Table 6.1 Components of Clinical Empathy

Components of Clinical Empathy	Description
Emotive	Experiencing another's emotions, also called affective empathy
Moral	Internal altruistic force that drives empathic action
Cognitive	Understanding another's state of mind, also called perspective-taking
Behavioral	Communicating understanding of another's perspective

Source: Adapted from J.M. Morse, G. Anderson, J.L. Bottorff, O. Yonge, B. O'Brien, S.M. Solberg, and K.H. McIlveen, "Exploring Empathy: A Conceptual Fit for Nursing Practice?" *J Nurs Scholarsh* 24, no. 4 (1992): 273–280, https://doi.org/10.1111/j.1547-5069.1992.tb00733.x. Used by permission.

response to convey understanding of another's perspective. Whereas emotive or moral empathy may be ingrained and difficult to train, cognitive and especially behavioral empathy, which is a driving force for effective communication in the clinic, are value-neutral and malleable.

Definitions of empathy, compassion, and sympathy

The concepts of empathy, compassion, and sympathy are defined and conceptualized in many different ways in the literature and are often used interchangeably.[39] To dispel any confusion, we view empathy in this book as a broad concept that drives the response of compassion. The cognitive aspect of empathy is necessary for the response of empathic concern, often referred to as *compassion,* which may lead to positive feelings and protect against burnout by fostering greater engagement with patients.[40] Sympathy is an interrelated concept referring to general *fellow feeling,* which has been viewed by some as deriving from empathy and by others as wholly separate from empathy. However, sympathy has been conceptualized as a self-orientated response that necessarily creates a divide between the observer and patient: the observer feels a sense of pity.[41] Therefore, using our definition of sympathy, it is not as useful a construct in the physician–patient relationship.

Tools to measure communication, empathy, and compassion

Multiple tools to measure the communication skills of physicians have been developed. Following the publication of the Gap–Kalamazoo Consensus Statement, the Gap–Kalamazoo Communication Skills Assessment Form was developed as a tool to assess physician–patient communication. The form consists of seven evidence-based "essential elements," or tasks, of effective physician–patient communication and provides skill competencies for each element, The Patient–Practitioner Orientation Scale is an 18-item measure designed to assess the patient-centeredness of communication. The Patient–Practitioner Orientation Scale contains two subscales: sharing and caring.

Tools to measure empathy have also been developed. Because empathy is a complex construct without a clear, universal definition, measuring empathy is a challenging task. However, there exists a long history of developing tools to assess empathy. Tools such as the Hogan Empathy Scale, developed in 1969, or the Interpersonal Reactivity Index (IRI), developed in 1983, have been frequently used as assessment tools for research. Tools to assess empathy can be grouped as

- Self-report measures, such as the Toronto Empathy Questionnaire.
- Behavioral measures such as picture-viewing paradigms.
- Physiological measures such as heart rate and skin conductance, as used by Riess.

However, all of these tools were developed for administration to the general public and are not designed for specific use in the clinical setting.

Recognizing the need for a measure of clinical empathy in medical education, Hojat and other scholars at Thomas Jefferson University developed the Jefferson Scale in 2002. It focuses on the cognitive aspect of empathy, and consists of 20 statements to which responders rank their agreement on a 7-point Likert scale. Examples of statements include "My understanding of how my patients and their families feel do not influence medical or surgical treatment" and "I try to think like my patients to render better care."

Neuroscience of empathy

Unlike psychological concepts, which can prove highly variable, hard to observe and reproduce, and easily affected by situational factors and individual psyche, studying the underlying neurological processes of empathy using functional magnetic resonance imaging (fMRI) is an emerging discipline in neurobiology. This research is very promising, because if we can understand how components of empathy are produced in the brain, we could then work toward strategies to cultivate those neural pathways. However, because the brain is not a modular system and many different regions of the brain light up when subjects experience empathy, it is difficult to pinpoint the exact neural pathways involved.

The study of the neurobiology of empathy was advanced by Rizzolatti and coauthors when they posited their theory of mirror neurons that fire both when one is performing an activity and when one is watching others perform it.[42] They studied macaque monkeys and observed that certain parts of the brain would light up when the monkeys performed an action and when they observed a similar action made by another monkey or the experimenter. Preston and de Waal performed the first fMRI experiments on humans regarding empathy and found that certain regions of the brain—specifically, the anterior insula, anterior cingulate cortex, and inferior frontal cortex— would fire when subjects were experiencing a strong emotion and when they observed another person experiencing the same emotion.[43] A separate study found that people who had higher self-reported empathy exhibited stronger activation in the mirror neurons believed to be associated with emotions, adding credence to the theory that mirror neurons are involved in empathy.[44] Singer and coauthors compared brain activity when subjects experienced pain to brain activity when subjects were made aware that a loved one (in the same room) was experiencing a similar pain.[45] The bilateral anterior insula, rostral anterior cingulate cortex, brainstem, and cerebellum were all activated during both painful and empathic events. Figure 6.2 shows an fMRI image of the regions of the brain implicated in empathy.

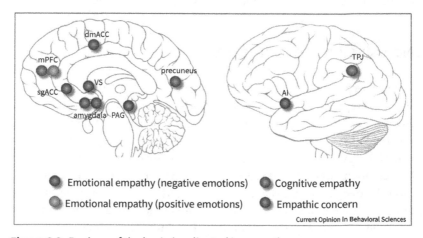

Figure 6.2 Regions of the brain implicated in empathy.

Table 6.2 Mapping of Empathic Responses using fMRI

Type of Empathic Response	Characterized By	Regions of the Brain That Are Implicated
Empathic distress	Negative feelings (e.g., stress, anxiety, burnout); leads to nonsocial behavior	Insula and anterior middle cingulate cortex
Empathic concern/ compassion	Positive feelings (e.g. love, caring); could protect against burnout, leads to prosocial behavior	Medial orbitofrontal cortex, dorsal medial prefrontal cortex, and ventral striatum

Recent literature has focused on mapping the two different responses to empathy in the brain—empathic distress and empathic concern—which we also refer to as compassion. A study found that these processes were associated with activity in different regions in the brain.[46] While the empathic distress response was localized to premotor and somatosensory regions involved in representing both one's own and others' bodily states, the empathic concern response was preferentially implicated in the ventromedial prefrontal cortex, medial orbitofrontal cortex, and ventral striatum, which have been found to drive prosocial behavior. Empathic concern/compassion was also related to activity in the septal area of the basal forebrain, which has been shown through fMRI studies to be implicated in feelings of affiliative emotion,[47] trust,[48] and charitable donation.[49] The empathic distress and compassion responses are described in Table 6.2.

Can empathy and compassion be developed?

Children typically begin to develop empathy very early on, usually around the age of one or two. Precursors for empathy are noted 18 to 72 hours after birth in terms of a newborn responding more intensely to the sound of another infant crying than other noises.[50] As infants begin to develop differentiation between self and other, they naturally begin to develop the ability to engage in perspective-taking. However, are physicians able to learn empathy long after these developmental processes occur?

Many physicians often claim that empathy cannot be taught, but evidence shows that there are components of empathy that can be developed through training. Within the framework of the Morse model, it seems likely that emotive and moral empathy are hardwired, but the cognitive and behavioral aspects of empathy—or how we develop an understanding of other's emotions and shape our actions accordingly—are malleable. Crucially, this indicates that compassion, which stems largely from cognitive empathy, is trainable as well.[51] With a growing body of research supporting the efficacy of empathy training, initiatives to develop empathy and compassion in students and residents have arisen across the country. For example, Helen Riess developed a course called Empathetics required for all residents at Massachusetts General Hospital and other Harvard Medical School teaching hospitals.[52] Stanford University Medical School developed the Standardized Patient Program in which medical students develop empathy skills by interacting with actors in a simulated clinical environment as early as the first quarter of medical school.[53] Initiatives for compassion training—for example, through the Human Kindness curriculum at the University of California Irvine Medical School—are beginning to take hold.[54] Even as medical schools move toward a holistic review process for admissions and select for communication and empathy skills in their students, medical schools and residency programs are recognizing the value of fostering these skills in training. Learners interested in expanding their empathetic and communication skills in general may consider the exercises and practices presented in Box 6.2.

Why are communication and empathy so important?

The racial and cultural diversity of America's patient population places additional demands on a physician's communication and empathy skills, particularly in combatting implicit bias. In their interactions with African-American patients, American physicians have been shown to exhibit less nonverbal attention, empathy, courtesy, and information giving; to adopt a more "narrowly biomedical" communication style; to spend less time providing health education, chatting, and answering questions; and to be more verbally dominant and exhibit more negative emotional tone than with

---

Box 6.2 Ways to Retain and Enhance Empathy

- Communication skills training
- Self-awareness, emotional recognition
- Analyzing encounters with patients
- Role-playing, especially of physician–patient interactions
- Exposure to positive role models
- Shadowing patients
- Experiencing hospitalization
- Studying literature and arts
- Watching theatrical performances
- Improving narrative skills—narrative medicine
- Small-group discussions
- Self-care, attention to own happiness
- Mindfulness, meditation
- Practice identifying facial expressions/nonverbal communications

---

white patients.[55] Empathy becomes, at once, more urgent and more difficult due to unconscious bias.

In addition, communication skills and empathy are purported to decline as medical students progress through their medical education and clinical practice. It is helpful to consider the decline as occurring in two distinct phases: in the medical education process and, later, in the physician's career. In the medical education process, the decline is likely due to the overwhelming volume of information that must be processed and retained. In their article on the helplessness that clinicians sometimes feel, Larsson and Stern cite the "classic 'emergency room panic' of the newly minted medical graduate faced with an acutely ill patient."[56] Hojat and coauthors also point to poor workplace environment and treatment from superiors that set expectations and norms for how physicians should behave, especially during residency. Later in the physician's career, however, studies have shown that insufficient empathy is caused by helplessness. The National Academy of Medicine cited a "perceived loss of control and meaning at work" as a contributing factor to burnout in working physicians.[57p313] The *Handbook of*

Stress, Theoretical and Clinical Aspects supports this theory, showing that physicians who display high levels of idealism and commitment are most apt to burnout (see Chapter 10 of this volume).[58]

However, burnout is closely related to the concept of compassion fatigue, which refers to emotional exhaustion that leads to an inability to empathize or feeling compassion for others. Compassion fatigue is derived from empathic distress, while compassion actually protects against compassion fatigue. Physicians who incorporate compassion into their care may engage in more meaningful empathic connections and find greater satisfaction in their work.[59]

Chapter Quick Summary

- The interpersonal skills of communication, empathy, and compassion are vital for physicians in today's healthcare environment.
- Effective communication benefits both patients and physicians, and physician reimbursement and online ratings take into account communication abilities.
- Patient-centered care requires effective communication. Elements of effective communication include active listening and the apology.
- Empathy is defined generally as the ability to understand and share the feelings of others. It is linked with increased patient satisfaction, interpersonal trust between patients and physicians, adherence with physicians' recommendations, decreased patient anxiety and distress, better clinical outcomes, decreased physician burnout, and lower risk of malpractice suits.
- Empathy has emotive, moral, cognitive, and behavioral components.
- The neurological processes of empathy are highlighted including the regions of the brain that are implicated.
- Compassion is an empathic response that may lead to greater engagement and protect against compassion fatigue and burnout.
- Components of empathy and compassion can be developed, and medical schools and residency programs are beginning to adopt curricula for empathy and compassion training.

Resources

Academy of Communication in Healthcare. "Resources: Videos." https://www.achonline.org/Resources/Videos

Joint Commission on Hand-Offs. "Inadequate Hand-Off Communication." *Sentinel Event Alert.* September 12, 2017. https://www.jointcommission.org/-/media/tjc/documents/resources/patient-safety-topics/sentinel-event/sea_58_hand_off_comms_9_6_17_final_(1).pdf

Makoul, G. "Essential Elements of Communication in Medical Encounters: The Kalamazoo Consensus Statement." *Acad Med* 76, no. 4 (April 2001): 390–393. https://doi.org/10.1097/00001888-200104000-00021

Mazzolini, C., and F.M. Cummings. "Malpractice and Apology Laws: The Pros and Cons" [Video]. *Medical Economics.* January 14, 2020. https://www.medicaleconomics.com/videos-medical-economics/malpractice-and-apology-laws-pros-and-cons

MedEdPortal. [Home page]. https://www.mededportal.org/

Morton, H. "Medical Professional Apology Statutes." *National Conference of State Legislatures.* December 11, 2018. https://www.ncsl.org/research/financial-services-and-commerce/medical-professional-apologies-statutes.aspx

NEJM Knowledgment+. "Exploring the ACGME Core Competencies (Part 1 of 7)." June 2, 2016. https://knowledgeplus.nejm.org/blog/exploring-acgme-core-competencies/

Riess, H. *Empathy Effect: Seven Neuroscience-Based Keys for Transforming the Way We Live, Love, Work, and Connect Across Differences.* Boulder, CO: Sounds True, 2018.

Spandorfer, J., C. Pohl, T. Nasca, S.L. Rattner, eds. *Professionalism in Medicine: A Case-Based Guide for Medical Students.* Cambridge: Cambridge University Press, 2010.

STEPS Forward. [Home page]. *American Medical Association.* https://edhub.ama-assn.org/steps-forward

VitalTalk. [Home page]. https://www.vitaltalk.org/

References

1. Addams, A.N., R.B. Bletzinger, H.M. Sondheimer, S.E. White, and L.M. Johnson. *Roadmap to Diversity: Integrating Holistic Review Practices into Medical School Admission Processes.* Washington, DC: Association of American Medical Colleges, 2010.

2. Hall, J.A., D.L. Roter, and C.S. Rand. "Communication of Affect between Patient and Physician." *J Health Soc Behav* 22, no. 1 (1981): 18–30. https://doi.org/10.2307/2136365.

3. Kaplan, S.H., S. Greenfield, and J.E. Ware. "Assessing the Effects of Physician-Patient Interactions on the Outcomes of Chronic Disease." *Med Care* 27, no. 3 (1989): S110–S127.

4. Ha J.F., and N. Longnecker. "Doctor–Patient Communication: A Review." *Ochsner J* 10, no. 1 (2010): 38–43.

5. Adamy, J. "US Ties Hospital Payments to Making Patients Happy." *The Wall Street Journal*. October 14, 2012. https://www.wsj.com/articles/SB10000872396390443890304578010264156073132

6. Zgierska, A., D. Rabago, and M.M. Miller. "Impact of Patient Satisfaction Ratings on Physicians and Clinical Care." *Patient Prefer Adher* 8 (2014): 437–446.

7. Boissy, A., A.K. Windover, D. Bokar, M. Karafa, K. Neuendorf, R.M. Frankel, J. Merlino, and M.B. Rothberg. "Communication Skills Training for Physicians Improves Patient Satisfaction." *J Gen Inter Med* 31, no. 7 (2016): 755–761. https://doi.org/10.1007/s11606-016-3597-2

8. Hanauer, D.A., K. Zheng, D.C. Singer, A. Gebremariam, and M.M. Davis. "Public Awareness, Perception, and Use of Online Physician Rating Sites." *JAMA* 311, no. 7 (2014): 734–735. https://doi.org/10.1001/jama.2013.283194

9. Okike, K., T.K. Peter-Bibb, K.C. Xie, and O.N. Okike. "Association Between Physician Online Rating and Quality of Care." *J Med Internet Res* 18, no. 12 (2016): e324. https://doi.org/10.2196/jmir.6612

10. Becker, G., D.E. Kempf, C.J. Xander, F. Momm, M. Olschewski, and H.E. Blum. "Four Minutes for a Patient, Twenty Seconds for a Relative: An Observational Study at a University Hospital." *BMC Health Serv Res* 10, no. 94 (2010): 1–9.

11. Tongue, J.R., H.R. Epps, and L.L. Forese. "Communication Skills." *AAOS Instr Cours Lec* 54 (2005): 3–9.

12. CRICO Strategies. "Malpractice Risks in Communication Failures: 2015 Annual Benchmarking Report." 2015. https://www.rmf.harvard.edu/Malpractice-Data/Annual-Benchmark-Reports/Risks-in-Communication-Failures

13. Panesar, S.S., D. deSilva, A. Carson-Stevens, K.M. Cresswell, S.A. Salvilla, S.P. Slight, S. Javad, G. Netuveli, I. Larizgoitia, L.J. Donaldson, D.W. Bates, and A. Sheikh. "How Safe Is Primary Care? A Systematic Review." *BMJ Qual Safe* 25, no. 7 (2016): 544–553. https://doi.org/10.1136/bmjqs-2015-004178

14. Lahue, B.J., B. Pyenson, K. Iwasaki, H.E. Blumen, S. Forray, and J.M. Rothschild. "National Burden of Preventable Adverse Drug Events Associated with Inpatient

Injectable Medications: Healthcare and Medical Professional Liability Costs." *Amer Health Drug Ben* 5, no. 7 (2012): 1–10.

15. Lindquist, L.A., A. Yamahiro, A. Garrett, C. Zei, and J.M. Feinglass. "Primary Care Physician Communication at Hospital Discharge Reduces Medication Discrepancies." *J Hosp Med* 8, no. 12 (2013): 672–677. https://doi.org/10.1002/jhm.2098

16. "Inadequate Hand-off Communication." *Sentinel Event Alert* 58 (2017): 1–6. https://www.jointcommission.org/resources/patient-safety-topics/sentinel-event/sentinel-event-alert-newsletters/sentinel-event-alert-58-inadequate-hand-off-communication/

17. Ong, L.M., J.C. de Haes, A.M. Hoos, and F.B. Lammes. "Doctor–Patient Communication: A Review of the Literature." *Soc Sci Med* 40, no. 7 (1995): 903–918.

18. VandeKieft, G.K. "Breaking Bad News." *Am Fam Physician* 64, no. 12 (2001): 1975–1978.

19. Orlander, J.D., B.G. Fincke, D. Hermanns, and G.A. Johnson. "Medical Residents' First Clearly Remembered Experiences of Giving Bad News." *J Gen Inter Med* 17, no. 11 (2002): 825–831. https://doi.org/10.1046/j.1525-1497.2002.10915.x

20. Schmid Mast, M., A. Kindlimann, and W. Langewitz. "Recipients' Perspective on Breaking Bad News: How You Put It Really Makes a Difference." *Patient Educ Couns* 58, no. 3 (2005): 244–251. https://doi.org/10.1016/j.pec.2005.05.005

21. Monden, K.R., L. Gentry, T.R. Cox. "Delivering Bad News to Patients." *Baylor University Medical Center Proceedings* 29, no. 1 (2016): 101–102. https://doi.org/10.1080/08998280.2016.11929380

22. Baile, W.F., R. Buckman, R. Lenzi, G. Glober, E.A. Beale, and A.P. Kudelka. "SPIKES: A Six-step Protocol for Delivering Bad News: Application to the Patient with Cancer." *Oncologist* 5, no. 4 (2000): 302–311. https://doi.org/10.1634/theoncologist.5-4-302

23. Rabow, M.W., and S.J. McPhee. "Beyond Breaking Bad News: How to Help Patients Who Suffer." *Western J Med* 171, no. 4 (1999): 260–263.

24. Blumenthal-Barby, J.S., L. Loftis, C.L. Cummings, W. Meadow, M. Lemmon, P.A. Ubel, L. McCullough, E. Rao, and J.D. Lantos. "Should Neonatologists Give Opinions Withdrawing Life-sustaining Treatment?" *Pediatrics* 138, no. 6 (2016): e20162585. https://doi.org/10.1542/peds.2016-2585

25. Bryan, C.S. *Osler: Inspirations from a Great Physician*. New York: Oxford University Press, 1997.

26. Singh Ospina, N., K.A. Phillips, R. Rodriguez-Gutierrez, A. Castaneda-Guarderas, M.R. Gionfriddo, M.E. Branda, and V.M. Montori. "Eliciting the Patient's Agenda- Secondary Analysis of Recorded Clinical Encounters." *J Gen Inter Med* 34, no. 1 (2019): 36–40. https://doi.org/10.1007/s11606-018-4540-5

27. "The Michigan Model: Medical Malpractice and Patient Safety at Michigan Medicine | Michigan Medicine." *Michigan Medicine.* July 6, 2020. https://www.uofmhealth.org/michigan-model-medical-malpractice-and-patient-safety-umhs

28. American Medical Association. "AMA Code of Medical Ethics Opinion 8.6 Promoting Patient Safety." https://www.ama-assn.org/system/files/2020-12/code-of-medical-ethics-chapter-8.pdf

29. Jackson, J.L., and K. Kroenke. "Difficult Patient Encounters in the Ambulatory Clinic: Clinical Predictors and Outcomes." *Arch Inter Med* 159, no. 10 (1999): 1069–1075. https://doi.org/10.1001/archinte.159.10.1069

30. Steinmetz, D., and H. Tabenkin. "The 'Difficult Patient' as Perceived by Family Physicians." *Fam Prac* 18, no. 5 (2001): 495–500. https://doi.org/10.1093/fampra/18.5.495

31. Hahn, S.R., K. Kroenke, R.L. Spitzer, D. Brody, J.B.W. Williams, M. Linzer, and F.V. deGruy. "The Difficult Patient." *J Gen Inter Med* 11, no. 1 (1996): 1–8. https://doi.org/10.1007/BF02603477

32. J. Manyika, M. Chui, M. Miremadi, J. Bughin, K. George, P.J. Willmott, and M. Dewhurst. "A Future that Works: Automation, Employment and Productivity." *McKinsey Global Institute.* January 2017. https://www.mckinsey.com/~/media/McKinsey/Featured%20Insights/Digital%20Disruption/Harnessing%20automation%20for%20a%20future%20that%20works/MGI-A-future-that-works_Executive-summary.pdf

33. Buro, J.S. "App Review Series: Doximity." *J Dig Imag* 32, no. 1 (2019): 1–5. https://doi.org/10.1007/s10278-018-0109-4

34. Decety, J., and A. Fotopoulou. "Why Empathy Has a Beneficial Impact on Others in Medicine: Unifying Theories." *Front Behav Neurosci* 8 (2015): 457. https://doi.org/10.3389/fnbeh.2014.00457.

35. Jamison, L. *The Empathy Exams: Essays.* Minneapolis, MN: Graywolf Press, 2014.

36. Morse, J.M., G. Anderson, J.L. Bottorff, O. Yonge, B. O'Brien, S.M. Solberg, and K.H. McIlveen. "Exploring Empathy: A Conceptual Fit for Nursing Practice?" *J Nurs Scholarship* 24, no. 4 (1992): 273–280. https://doi.org/10.1111/j.1547-5069.1992.tb00733.x

37. Shamay-Tsoory, S.G., J. Aharon-Peretz, and D. Perry. "Two Systems for Empathy: A Double Dissociation between Emotional and Cognitive Empathy in

Inferior Frontal Gyrus versus Ventromedial Prefrontal Lesions." *Brain* 132, no. 3 (2009): 617–627. https://doi.org/10.1093/brain/awn279

38. Halpern, J. "What is Clinical Empathy?" *J Gen Inter Med* 18, no. 8 (2003): 670–674. https://doi.org/10.1046/j.1525-1497.2003.21017.x

39. Jeffrey, D. "Empathy, Sympathy and Compassion in Healthcare: Is There a Problem? Is There a Difference? Does It Matter?" *J Royal Soc Med* 109, no. 12 (2016): 446–452. https://doi.org/10.1177/0141076816680120

40. Cameron, R.A., B.L. Mazer, J.M. DeLuca, S.G. Mohile, and R.M. Epstein. "In Search of Compassion: A New Taxonomy of Compassionate Physician Behaviours." *Health Expect* 18, no. 5 (2015): 1672–1685. https://doi.org/10.1111/hex.12160

41. Hojat, M., M.J. Vergare, K. Maxwell, G. Brainard, S.K. Herrine, G.A. Isenberg, J. Veloski, and J.S. Gonnella. "The Devil Is in the Third Year: A Longitudinal Study of Erosion of Empathy in Medical School." *Acad Med* 84, no. 9 (2009): 1182–1191. https://doi.org/10.1097/ACM.0b013e3181b17e55

42. Rizzolatti, G., L. Fadiga, V. Gallese, and L. Fogassi. "Premotor Cortex and the Recognition of Motor Actions." *Cog Brain Res* 3, no. 2 (1996): 131–141. https://doi.org/10.1016/0926-6410(95)00038-0

43. Preston, S.D., and F.B.M. de Waal. "Empathy: Its Ultimate and Proximate Bases." *Behav Brain Sci* 25, no. 1 (2002): 1–20. https://doi.org/10.1017/S0140525X02000018

44. Gazzola, V., L. Aziz-Zadeh, and C. Keysers. "Empathy and the Somatotopic Auditory Mirror System in Humans," *Curr Biol* 16, no. 18 (2006): 1824–1829. https://doi.org/10.1016/j.cub.2006.07.072

45. Singer, T., B. Seymour, J. O'Doherty, H. Kaube, R.J. Dolan, and C.D. Frith. "Empathy for Pain Involves the Affective but Not Sensory Components of Pain." *Science* 303, no. 5661 (2004): 1157–1162. https://doi.org/10.1126/science.1093535.

46. Ashar, Y.K., J.R. Andrews-Hanna, S. Dimidjian, and T.D. Wager. "Empathic Care and Distress: Predictive Brain Markers and Dissociable Brain Systems." *Neuron* 94, no. 6 (2017): 1263–1273. https://doi.org/10.1016/j.neuron.2017.05.014

47. Morelli, S.A., L.T. Rameson, and M.D. Lieberman. "The Neural Components of Empathy: Predicting Daily Prosocial Behavior." *Soc Cogn Affect Neur* 9, no. 1 (2014): 39–47. https://doi.org/10.1093/scan/nss088

48. Krueger, F., K. McCabe, J. Moll, N. Kriegeskorte, R. Zahn, M. Strenziok, A. Heinecke, and J. Grafman. "Neural Correlates of Trust," *P Natl Acad Sci U S A* 104, no. 50 (2007): 20084–20089. https://doi.org/10.1073/pnas.0710103104.

49. Moll, J., F. Krueger, R. Zahn, R., M. Pardini, R. de Oliveira-Souza, and J. Grafman. "Human Fronto–Mesolimbic Networks Guide Decisions about Charitable Donation." *P Natl Acad Sci USA* 103, no. 42 (2016): 15623–15628. https://doi.org/10.1073/pnas.0604475103

50. Martin G.B., and R.D. Clark. "Distress Crying in Neonates: Species and Peer Specificity." *Dev Psychol* 18, no. 1(1982): 3–9. https://doi.org/10.1037/0012-1649.18.1.3

51. Weng, H.Y., R.C. Lapate, D.E. Stodola, G.M. Rogers, and R.J. Davidson. "Visual Attention to Suffering after Compassion Training Is Associated with Decreased Amygdala Responses." *Front Psychology* 9 (2018). https://doi.org/10.3389/fpsyg.2018.00771

52. Riess, H., and G. Kraft-Todd. "E.M.P.A.T.H.Y.: A Tool to Enhance Nonverbal Communication between Clinicians and Their Patients." *Acad Med* 89, no. 8 (2014): 1108–1112. https://doi.org/10.1097/ACM.0000000000000287

53. Stuart, E., S. Bereknyei, M. Long, R. Blankenburg, V. Weak, and R. Garcia. "Standardized Patient Cases for Skill Building in Patient-Centered, Cross-Cultural Interviewing (Stanford Gap Cases)." *MedEdPORTAL* 8 (2012). https://doi.org/10.15766/mep_2374-8265.9133

54. Shapiro, J., J. Youm, A. Kheriaty, T. Pham, Y. Chen, and R. Clayma. "The Human Kindness Curriculum: An Innovative Preclinical Initiative to Highlight Kindness and Empathy in Medicine." *Ed Health* 32, no. 2 (2019): 53–61. https://doi.org/10.4103/efh.efh_133_18

55. Beach, M.C., S. Saha, P.T. Korthuis, V. Sharp, J. Cohn, I.B. Wilson, S. Eggly, L.A. Cooper, D. Roter, A. Sankar, and R. Moore. "Patient–Provider Communication Differs for Black Compared to White HIV-Infected Patients." *AIDS Behav* 15, no. 4 (2011): 805–811. https://doi.org/10.1007/s10461-009-9664-5

56. Larsson, E.W., and T.A. Stern. "Helplessness in the Helpers: Etiology and Management." *Pri Care Companion CNS Dis* 15, no. 6 (2013). https://doi.org/10.4088/PCC.13f01538

57. Dzau, V.J., D.G. Kirch, and T.J. Nasca. "To Care Is Human: Collectively Confronting the Clinician-Burnout Crisis." *New Engl J Med* 378, no. 4 (2018): 312–314. https://doi.org/10.1056/NEJMp1715127

58. Goldberger, L., and S. Breznitz. *Handbook of Stress: Theoretical and Clinical Aspects.* New York: Free Press, 1986.

59. Halpern, J. "What Is Clinical Empathy?" *J Gen Inter Med* 18, no. 8 (2003): 670–674. https://doi.org/10.1046/j.1525-1497.2003.21017.x

7
Developing Cultural Praxis

As medical professionals, you will encounter, treat, and work with patients of all cultures. Unlike in many other professions, practicing medicine often requires an intimate understanding of where a patient stands on many issues, ranging from opinions on animal product use to willingness to undergo certain kinds of surgeries. Patients' beliefs and attitudes are derived from their *culture*, defined as the "integrated pattern of thoughts, communications, actions, customs, beliefs, values, and institutions associated, wholly or partially, with racial, ethnic, or linguistic groups, as well as with religious, spiritual, biological, geographical, or sociological characteristics."[1p10] It is important to note that an individual's cultural identification may change over time.

Physicians have a responsibility to provide a high standard of care to all patients according to the ethical principle of justice, and care should not vary due to the cultural characteristics of patients, a concept referred to as health equity. Many of the current buzzwords in healthcare relate to this concept, such as multicultural health, cultural sensitivity, and unconscious bias. However, in our society, sociocultural determinants of health exist and health disparities continue to persist. Furthermore, physicians may inadvertently engage in a process of implicit, or unconscious bias, in which they may act unknowingly on the basis of socialized prejudices and stereotypes, which may manifest in the form of microaggressions.

The limits of cultural competence

In the 1990s, realizing the necessity of considering the individual social, cultural, and psychological needs of patients in delivering equitable care, medical education curricula began to shift toward a model of *cultural competence*. Cultural competence was first defined in 1989 by Terry Cross in his seminal work *Towards a Culturally Competent System of Care* as a "set of congruent behaviors, attitudes, and policies that come together in a system, agency or among professionals and enable that system, agency or those professions to work effectively in cross-cultural situations."[2p8] In 2003, the American Council for Graduate Medical Education, which accredits all graduate medical education programs in the United States, established six core competencies for program directors to teach and assess. Cultural competency is recognized as a component of the competencies of patient care, professionalism, and interpersonal and communication skills. In the common program requirements, the American Council for Graduate Medical Education states that "residents/fellows are expected to communicate effectively with patients, families, and the public, as appropriate across a broad range of socioeconomic and cultural backgrounds," as well as demonstrate a "sensitivity and responsiveness to a diverse patient population."[3]

Other associations followed suit. In 2004, the Liaison Committee on Medical Education, which accredits U.S. medical schools, stated that all medical students must demonstrate a standard level of cultural competence at graduation.[4] In 2013, the American Association of Medical Colleges established that cultural competence is one of the 15 core competencies necessary for entering medical students.[5] Clearly, the leaders in medical education have realized the importance of teaching about culture in the form of cultural competence training. Nevertheless, the term "cultural competence" indicates mastery: a finished process that does not need continued refinement through the process of lifelong learning. As a result, we believe that this term by itself is of questionable sufficiency to describe an ongoing process in medicine. For the purposes of this chapter, we will use the term cultural competence to describe the foundational set of knowledge, skills, and attitudes necessary for physicians to continue to develop a professional identity around social justice and health equity.

Cultural humility through the development of a critical consciousness

The concept of *cultural humility* was first defined by Melanie Tervalon and Jann Murray-Garcia in 1998 as an ongoing process of self-reflection in order to develop cultural awareness.[6] Cultural humility involves an internalization of a novel way of thinking about the world rather than mastery of a set of knowledge, skills, and attitudes vis-à-vis culture competence. The process of developing cultural humility incorporates tenets of professional identity formation and fits within the framework of lifelong learning. Crucially, cultural humility moves away from a paternalistic model and focuses on patient-centered care; the culturally humble physician understands that each patient possesses unique perspectives and desires that are socialized from their culture. By using patient-centered interviewing and active-listening strategies (see Chapter 6 of this volume), physicians are able to employ an open-minded attitude to understand the multifaceted components of each individual. Furthermore, physicians who engage in cultural humility understand that they cannot be fully informed about all cultures and strive not to make stereotypical assumptions. Instead, they let the patient lead and incorporate the information that patients share into the clinical decision-making process.

Arno Kumagai and colleagues suggested viewing cultural humility through the framework of developing a *critical consciousness*—of self, others, and the world.[7] The theory of critical consciousness, developed by Paulo Freire, posits that thinking individuals do not exist in a vacuum, but within the context of interaction with others.[8] Systems of power and inequity drive society and its interactions, and by developing critical consciousness, one is able to develop an awareness of these systems. Other authors, identifying the long-standing racial disparities in law enforcement—recently highlighted by the death of Freddie Gray, George Floyd, Breonna Taylor, and Philando Castille—have recognized the need for formal medical education for social justice.[9] These authors suggest the concept of structural competency, which refers to examining forces that lead to inequity that are beyond the scope of the patient–physician relationship.

By developing a critical consciousness or developing structural competency, one becomes committed to social justice, which in the context of medicine is about providing equitable care to all members of society.[7] Through the process of developing a critical consciousness, or what Freire calls *conscientization*, one's beliefs and attitudes are fundamentally transformed and begin to shape one's actions. Similar to reaching the "is" stage of the amended Miller pyramid suggested by Cruess and Cruess (see Figure 1.1 in Chapter 1 of this volume), in which the physician has fully internalized their professional identity and lives it, physicians who undergo conscientization work to internalize the values of cultural humility. Particularly in today's healthcare environment, in which physicians feel the pressure of limited time to see patients, it is important that the process of cultural awareness and the actions derived from that awareness are automatic.

Cultural praxis as a means toward social justice and health equity

Freire suggested that the goal of developing a critical consciousness on a societal level is *praxis*, informed action committed to human well-being and uncovering truth. Awareness without action is insufficient. While action driven by cultural humility exists primarily in the interpersonal space of physician–patient interactions, if we are to view cultural humility within the context of conscientization, there must also be a component of praxis to combat health disparities at institutional and policy levels. We propose the term "cultural praxis," which encompasses the values of cultural awareness and cultural humility and includes informed action toward social justice. Cultural praxis involves participating in initiatives to spread awareness, incorporating policies to reduce systemic exclusion, and advocating for disadvantaged populations. By themselves, cultural competence and cultural humility are inadequate in medical education. Whereas others have suggested merging the concepts of cultural competence and cultural humility into a term called "cultural competemility," we propose instead the addition of "cultural praxis" as an additional stage in the continuum of cultural awareness, involving a transformation in beliefs and attitudes and actions at the individual, institutional, and policy levels that reflect it (see Figure 7.1).[10]

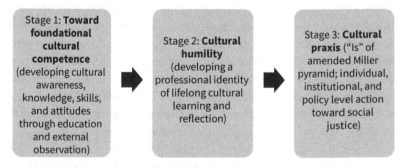

Figure 7.1 Developmental stages of cultural praxis. Stage 1: toward *foundational* cultural competence (developing cultural awareness, knowledge, skills, and attitudes through education and external observation) → Stage 2: cultural humility (developing a professional identity of lifelong cultural learning and reflection) → Stage 3: cultural praxis ("Is" of Miller pyramid; individual, institutional, and policy level action toward social justice).

Sociocultural determinants of health disparities

A compelling body of evidence shows that sociocultural determinants shape health outcomes. According to the World Health Organization, social determinants of health are the "conditions in which people are born, grow, work, live, and age, and the wider set of forces and systems shaping the conditions of daily life."[11] We believe that these conditions are more accurately described as the sociocultural determinants of health, as our conception of culture encompasses *the wider set of forces and systems shaping the conditions of daily life.* These sociocultural determinants of health work to create persistent disparities in healthcare between the overall population and certain vulnerable subpopulations, as distinguished by factors such as race, age, religion, and immigrant status. They work at micro, meso, and macro levels to influence health outcomes, as described by Dahlgren and Whitehead.[12] Not only is health influenced by genetics and individual lifestyle factors, but it is also derived from community influences, living and working conditions, and other economic and sociocultural factors. Figure 7.2 describes the Dahlgren–Whitehead rainbow model of social determinants of health.

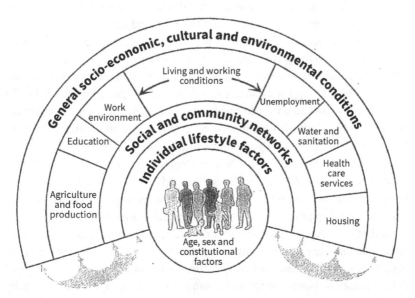

Figure 7.2   Dahlgren-Whitehead rainbow model of social determinants of health.

From G. Dahlgren and M. Whitehead, "Policies and Strategies to Promote Social Equity in Health (Stockholm, Sweden: Institute for Futures Studies, 1990), https://www.iffs.se/media/1326/20080109110739filmZ8UVQv2wQFShMRF6cuT.pdf. Used by permission.

Box 7.1 Statistics on Cultural Diversity in the United States, 2019

- Approximately 40 percent of Americans belong to a racial or ethnic minority population.[13]
- Approximately 51 percent of Americans are women.
- Roughly 26 percent of adult Americans have some sort of disability.[14]
- An estimated 84 percent of the population lives in urban areas, while 16 percent of the population lives in rural areas.[15]
- An estimated 4.5 percent of Americans identify as lesbian, gay, bisexual, or transgender.[16]

To better understand the context of health disparities, it is helpful to learn about the cultural diversity of the U.S. population (Box 7.1). Culture includes dimensions of race, ethnicity, age, ability, gender, sexual orientation, religion, geography, language, and socioeconomic status. The United States was built upon the values of egalitarianism and freedom and has espoused inclusive policies throughout its history. As a result, it has become a culturally pluralistic country, valuing the cultural identity of minority groups. However, cultural pluralism necessarily indicates that a dominant culture exists. In the context of healthcare, the existence of a dominant culture may lead to health disparities. By engaging in culturally respectful healthcare practices, we may strive toward cultural equity, in which the power dynamics that exist with the presence of a dominant group are reduced.

According to the Centers for Disease Control and Prevention, health disparities are "preventable differences in the burden of disease, injury, violence, or opportunities to achieve optimal health that are experienced by socially disadvantaged populations."[17] Health disparities adversely affect populations that experience systemic barriers to healthcare. For example, African American and Hispanic populations in the United States have lower rates of insurance coverage, constituting a barrier to access of care.[18] Sociocultural determinants of health—such as high-quality education, access to healthy foods, and safe housing—all contribute to health disparities (Box 7.2). One of the major goals of public health is health equity, or attainment of the highest level of health for all people. To achieve health equity, an awareness

Box 7.2 Examples of Racial and Ethnic Health Disparities

- The average waiting time for African Americans needing kidney transplants is almost twice as long as that of White patients.
- African American women with breast cancer are 67 percent more likely to die from the disease than are White women.
- The mortality rate for African American infants is almost 2.5 times greater than it is for White infants.
- Hispanic and African American youth are substantially more likely to die from diabetes than White youth.
- African American, Hispanic, and Native American physicians are much more likely than White physicians to practice in underserved communities and to treat larger numbers of minority patients, irrespective of income.
- African American and Hispanic physicians are more likely to provide care to the poor and those on Medicaid. (This also holds true for female physicians.)
- Racial and ethnic minority patients who have a choice are more likely to select healthcare professionals of their own racial or ethnic background.
- Racial and ethnic minority patients are generally more satisfied with their care, and are more likely to report receiving higher-quality care, when treated by a health professional of their own racial or ethnic background.

Adapted from Health Professionals for Diversity Coalition, https://www.rasmussen.edu/degrees/nursing/blog/lack-of-cultural-diversity-in-healthcare/, and CDC Vital Signs Report, https://www.cdc.gov/minorityhealth/publications/index.html.

of the existence of health disparities must first be obtained. Then, action at all levels—interpersonal, institutional, and policy—must be taken to eliminate disparities.

The COVID-19 pandemic has put health disparities in sharp focus. Current data suggest that there is a disproportionate burden of illness and death on racial and ethnic minority groups. From data collected in New York

City on COVID-19 deaths, there was a stark discrepancy in death rates among Black/African Americans (92.3 deaths per 100,000 population) and Hispanic/Latinos (74.3) as compared to Whites (45.2) or Asians (34.5). The Centers for Disease Control and Prevention cites differences in living conditions, work circumstances, and underlying health conditions and lower access to care as some of the probable systemic causes for these disparities.[19] Another potential reason for why these disparities continue to persist is because medical education and research largely focuses on the dominant power group. For example, dermatology textbooks often only describe how certain conditions present for the white population, rather than accounting for racial differences.

Engaging in cultural praxis through critical consciousness empowers physicians to develop awareness of the systems of power and control that lead to inequity in healthcare. Using this awareness, physicians have a responsibility not only to deliver more equitable, individualized, patient-centered care, but also engage in praxis to address systemic issues at the meso and macro levels.

Hospitals and health systems spend $782 billion annually, employ more than 5.6 million people, and hold investment portfolios of more than $400 billion.[20] Compared to other developed countries, the United States spends far less on social care compared to healthcare. Institutional and systemic policies are long-established, and the paradigms of healthcare in the United States are difficult to change overnight. The initiative to address social determinants of health by Healthy People 2020[21] is a step in the right direction, but as culturally respectful physicians, we ought to engage in continued discourse and actions to work toward health equity.

Race and ethnicity of the physician workforce versus the general population

The American Association of Medical Colleges found that among active physicians, 56.2 percent identified as White, 17.1 percent identified as Asian, 5.8 percent identified as Hispanic, and 5.0 percent identified as Black or African American; 13.7 percent of active physicians identified as unknown.[22] According to the U.S. Census Bureau estimates from 2019, 76.5 percent of the general population is White, 5.9 percent Asian, 18.3 percent Hispanic or Latino, and 13.4 percent Black or African American.[13] The underrepresentation of the Hispanic and Black population in the physician workforce is striking.

Critical consciousness indicates that these discrepancies have systemic roots. For example, even the Flexner Report—which transformed the paradigms of medical education and training and has largely been a force for improving healthcare—has had wide-ranging impacts on perpetuating racial injustice in healthcare.[23] Flexner wrote in his report that African American physicians should be relegated to secondary roles and serving exclusively other African Americans. In addition, the Flexner Report caused five of seven historically Black medical schools to close down, decreasing the accessibility of the profession for the Black/African American population. Indeed, in 1910, when the Flexner Report was published, African Americans comprised 2.5 percent of the physician workforce, but about a hundred years later, in 2008, while the Black population increased, they still only comprised 2.2 percent of it.[24] Only with the recent incorporation of admissions policies to decrease exclusion and allow for equal opportunity has the percentage of Black physicians risen to 5.0 percent in 2019. Further change, driven by cultural praxis, is necessary to address these and other issues of inequity.

Strategies to develop cultural praxis

Strategies to develop cultural praxis are similar to those used to develop a professional identity. Because developing cultural praxis through critical consciousness involves a transformation and internalization of beliefs, engaging in the reflective process is necessary. When turning a critical gaze to one's beliefs, attitudes, and experiences and questioning one's world view through learning the narratives of others and engaging in clinical experiences, one may be confronted with cognitive disequilibrium. By resolving cognitive disequilibrium, learners may move through the stages of cultural development (see Chapter 2 of this volume).

It is also important to recognize that medical learners inherently enjoy privileged status due to their educational background. In addition, many medical learners may enjoy the privileges of youth, socioeconomic status, and racial/ethnic background, among others. By reflecting on the stories of people of different cultures, medical learners may learn to advocate and care for those who are different from them.

Although physicians may not intend to treat their patients differently, an important concept to consider is implicit bias. Through the process of socialization, all people develop biases, typically reflecting in-group preference and out-group exclusion. And these biases, however unconscious, may affect patient care. A study of physician implicit bias found that physicians had no explicit preference for White versus Black patients, but had implicit biases favoring White patients and held stereotypes that Black patients are less cooperative.[25] Furthermore, these implicit biases may lead to differences in treatment. As physicians, we must strive to abide by the principle of justice. By learning and reflecting on the stories of others, we work towards empathy for all of our patients.

Guidelines for implementing cultural praxis: the National CLAS Standards

The U.S. Department of Health and Human Services Office of Minority Health in 2000 first developed the National Standards for Culturally and Linguistically Appropriate Services in Health and Health Care (National CLAS Standards), which are a set of mandates, recommendations, and guidelines.[26] In 2010, the Department of Health and Human Services Office of Minority Health launched the National CLAS Standards Enhancement Initiative to update these standards to reflect more recent research, expand their scope, and account for the changing landscape of healthcare with respect to new legislation such as the Affordable Care Act. The Enhanced National CLAS Standards were published in 2013. These standards represent a more comprehensive view of health and culture and place emphasis on the shared responsibility of healthcare organizations and providers to work together to implement them. The Enhanced National CLAS Standards are organized around one principle standard—to "provide care and services responsive to diverse cultural health beliefs and practices, preferred languages, health literacy, and other communication needs"—and 14 other standards that are organized into three main themes: (i) governance, leadership and workforce; (ii) communication and language assistance; and (iii) engagement, continuous improvement, and accountability. By satisfying each of these 14 other standards, the principle standard can be met, advancing health equity, improving quality of care, and helping to eliminate health disparities. Therefore, the National CLAS Standards serve as a practical guide for implementing cultural praxis (see Table 7.1).

Table 7.1 The Enhanced National Standards for Culturally and Linguistically Appropriate Services in Health and Healthcare

Standards	Description
Principal standard	1. Provide care and services responsive to diverse cultural health beliefs and practices, preferred languages, health literacy, and other communication needs.
Governance, leadership, and workforce	2. Support organizational governance and leadership that promotes CLAS and health equity. 3. Support a culturally and linguistically diverse governance, leadership, and workforce. 4. Continually educate and train governance, leadership, and workforce in culturally and linguistically appropriate policies and practices.
Communication and language assistance	5. Offer language assistance to individuals who have limited English proficiency at no cost. 6. Inform all individuals of the availability of language assistance services in their preferred language, verbally and in writing. 7. Ensure the competence of individuals providing language assistance, avoiding use of untrained individuals and/or minors as interpreters. 8. Provide easy-to-understand print and multimedia materials and signage in the languages commonly used by the service population.
Engagement, continuous improvement, and accountability	9. Establish culturally and linguistically appropriate goals, policies, and management accountability. 10. Conduct ongoing assessments of the organization's CLAS-related activities and integrate CLAS-related measures into quality improvement. 11. Collect and maintain accurate and reliable demographic data to monitor and evaluate CLAS impact on health equity and outcomes and to inform service delivery. 12. Conduct assessments of community health assets and needs; use these assessments to plan and implement services that respond to the cultural and linguistic diversity of the service population. 13. Partner with the community to design, implement, and evaluate cultural and linguistic appropriateness. 14. Create conflict and grievance resolution processes that are culturally and linguistically appropriate. 15. Communicate the organization's progress in implementing and sustaining CLAS.

Note: CLAS = culturally and linguistically appropriate services.

From *National CLAS Standards* (Washington, DC: U.S. Department of Health and Human Services, 2013).

Special consideration for cultural praxis

One of the most difficult times to provide culturally aware care is at the end of life. There are three dimensions of end-of-life care that vary culturally: communication of bad news, locus of decision-making, and advance directives. Some cultures prefer that physicians do not disclose bad news and that decisions about end-of-life care be made with family members rather than themselves.[27] Many cultures defer end-of-life decision-making entirely to the physician. Some cultures insist that everything must be done to save a patient in the final stages of life, even when palliative care may provide a better end-of-life experience than invasive treatments. Action driven by cultural praxis in these circumstances calls for treating patients as individuals and considering the unique priorities of the patient and/or their family. Consider and reflect on the case study in Box 7.3, which describes a challenging situation in end-of-life care.

When linguistic barriers with patients exist, effective communication is challenging, and employing cultural praxis is recommended. Much of the U.S. population is limited English proficient (LEP), self-identifying as speaking English less than "very well." According to the Migration Policy Institute, while 64.7 million people aged five and older in the United States spoke a language other than English at home in 2015, only 60 percent of them were fully proficient in English.[28] LEP is a significant barrier to medical comprehension, increases the risk of adverse medication reactions, and increases the likelihood of being readmitted to the hospital within 30 days.[29] In medically adverse events, it was found that 46.8 percent of LEP cases result in moderate physical harm or worse, compared to 24.4 percent in English-speaking patients.[30]

Issues associated with treating patients with LEP can be addressed through the use of language services, including professional translators. Often, there are barriers to using translators due to availability, time constraints, or convenience. However, use of a professional translator has been shown to improve medical care in factors including medical comprehension, healthcare utilization, patient satisfaction, and clinical outcomes. If translators are inaccessible, ad hoc interpreters may be incorporated—including nonprofessionally trained interpreters such as friends, family members, or hospital staff—who can translate for physician and patient communications. However, using ad hoc interpreters can be tricky considering the risk that

Box 7.3 Patient Case Study in End-of-Life Care

Mr. K is a 68-year-old Japanese American man who has smoked one pack a day for 30 years. He has previously been diagnosed with severe chronic obstructive pulmonary disease. During a visit to the hospital for chest pain, a chest X-ray and computed tomography scan reveal the presence of lung cancer. Mr. K's wife admits that he has been very weak and is unable to walk or eat without pain. Mr. K's primary care physician wants to refer him to hospice care, but Mr. K insists that his son, who lives in another state, make the decision for him.

Mr. K's primary care physician calls the son on the phone, and the son agrees that his father should be provided with hospice care. However, he insists that the father not learn about his terminal illness. He insists that talking to his father about death will only lead to undue emotional burden. He also states that he and his family are responsible in their culture for "protecting him." The father does not participate in the conversation and has no advance directives.

Soon after, Mr. K admits to the hospital with severe pneumonia. Mr. K is barely conscious, and breathing is slow and irregular. His son, who had since moved in to take care of his father, asks if a feeding tube can be put in and considers aggressive treatment. Mr. K's wife does not want to see Mr. K suffer any further. After a long discussion with the physician, they both eventually agree that Mr. K is dying and agree to allow him to die with comfort measures. Mr. K dies within 10 hours of admission.

Opportunities for Reflection
- Describe ways that that the issue of informed consent can be approached while being culturally respectful.
- Should the physician have approached Mr. K to further assess his preference for learning about his medical condition?
- What are some other questions the physician could ask?

they may not have appropriate training and could relay incorrect information to either parties. The National CLAS Standards advise organizations to offer language assistance at no cost to individuals who have LEP. Healthcare organizations should be sure to inform individuals of these services and provide print materials in languages commonly used by the populations in their service area.

Some communication guidelines for talking to patients with different languages include making sure that information is clear, avoiding humor or sarcasm, speaking slowly, and avoiding jargon. Patients with a language issue—or those with a different cultural approach to healthcare—may not be comfortable admitting that they have not understood all of the information presented, or they may simply not realize that they do not have as good of a handle on their treatment as they think. One common technique for confirming comprehension is the "teach-back technique," which consists of asking the patient to present the information as they understand it, so that the physician may determine understanding. Examples of questions that the physician may ask include "How are you going to take your medications this week?" or "I want to make sure I've been clear, can you explain back to me what I've just told you?" Using these questions after each topic serves to ensure that patients are able to grasp the concepts discussed.

Universal values

Any method of culturally sensitive care must include the understanding that there are aspects of human attitudes and beliefs that are cross-cultural. Respect is one value that is generally consistent among cultures, particularly in professional settings. However, respect extends beyond mere manners. Physicians and patients must be able to accept each other's differing viewpoints and cultures and acknowledge that they may be wrong. This type of respect not only helps solidify the patient–physician relationship but can also improve outcomes.

A desire for effective communication of emotions is another aspect of the human experience that is cross-cultural. Although different cultures have their own nuances to communicating emotion, evidence suggests that the six universal emotions—which include disgust, sadness, happiness, fear, anger, and surprise—are shared. Medical professionals should be aware not only of the way in which they communicate these emotions but also their nonverbal communication: posture, physical contact, and eye contact can also send signals about focus and importance to patients of many cultures. Make sure to send the signal that you are engaged with your patient. If you must add to electronic medical records yourself in the presence of the patient, make sure that this is made clear to them and that they still have your full attention.

Empathy is another universal human value (see Chapter 6 of this volume). Expressing understanding of a patient's pain and suffering can impact the physician–patient relationship, medical outcomes, and the physician preferences of patients. Learning to develop empathy for those who are different from you and whose experiences are less familiar to you is a crucial, cross-cultural tool for providing healthcare to all patients.

Many ethical values are, more or less, universal, such as "Do no harm," "Treat your patient as you would want yourself to be treated," and "Allow the patient to make decisions about their medical care." For care to be patient-centered, patients must be able to choose their course of treatment after being offered all relevant information by their caretakers. If patients decide that they do not want to be responsible for making decisions about their care, the principle of autonomy also allows patients to transfer their ability of choice onto their physician, or onto a member of their family or trusted friend. The disease process is, itself, exhausting and emotionally draining, and some patients may decide that the burden of managing their own care is not one that they wish to shoulder during this difficult period in their lives.

Chapter Quick Summary

- Culture includes dimensions of race, ethnicity, age, ability, gender, sexual orientation, religion, geography, language, and socioeconomic status.
- Cultural praxis encompasses the values of cultural awareness, cultural competence, and cultural humility.
- Developing cultural praxis comes from the development of a critical consciousness and drives informed action.
- Sociocultural determinants of health exist and contribute to health disparities.
- One of the tenets of medical professionalism is to practice cultural praxis, working towards social justice and health equity for all patients.

Resources

Acholonu, R.G., T.E. Cook, R.O. Roswell, and R.E. Greene. "Microaggressions in medical education." *MedEd Portal*. July 31, 2020. https://doi.org/10.15766/mep_2374-8265.10969

Association of American Medical Colleges. "Tool for Assessing Cultural Competence Training (TACCT)." https://www.aamc.org/what-we-do/mission-areas/diversity-inclusion/tool-for-assessing-cultural-competence-training

Bassett, M. "Why Your Doctor Should Care about Social Justice." *TEDMed2015*. November 2015. https://www.ted.com/talks/mary_bassett_why_your_doctor_should_care_about_social_justice#t-525267

"CREST Provides Cultural Respect Simulation Training." *Healthsimulation.com*. https://www.healthysimulation.com/8963/crest-provides-cultural-respect-simulation-training/

Diversity and Inclusion, Cornell Certificate Program. [Home page]. *eCornell*. https://www.ecornell.com/certificates/leadership-and-strategic-management/diversity-and-inclusion/

Health Equity. [Home page]. Centers for Disease Control and Prevention. https://www.cdc.gov/healthequity/index.html

Healthy People 2030. [Home page]. *Office of Disease Prevention and Health Promotion*. https://www.healthypeople.gov/

Hook, J.N., D.E. Davis, J. Owen, E.E. Worthington, and, S.O. Utsey. "Cultural Humility: Measuring Openness to Culturally Diverse Clients." *J Couns Psychol* 60, no. 3 (2013): 353–366. https://doi.org/10.1037/a003259

National Center for Cultural Competence. [Home page]. *Georgetown University*. https://nccc.georgetown.edu/

References

1. U.S. Department of Health and Human Services. "National Standards for Culturally and Linguistically Appropriate Services in Health and Health Care: A Blueprint for Advancing and Sustaining CLAS Policy and Practice." April 2013. https://www.thinkculturalhealth.hhs.gov/assets/pdfs/EnhancedCLASStandardsBlueprint.pdf
2. Cross, T.L. B.J. Bazron, K.W. Dennis, and M.R. Isaacs. "Towards a Culturally Competent System of Care: A Monograph on Effective Services for Minority

Children Who Are Severely Emotionally Disturbed." *CASSP Technical Assistance Center, Georgetown University Child Development Center.* May 1989. https://files.eric.ed.gov/fulltext/ED330171.pdf

3. Accreditation Council for Graduate Medical Education. "ACGME Common Program Requirements." 2019. https://www.acgme.org/What-We-Do/Accreditation/Common-Program-Requirements

4. Liaison Committee on Medical Education. "Functions and Structure of a Medical School." 2004. https://lcme.org/publications/

5. Association of American Medical Colleges. "Core Competencies for Entering Medical Students." https://www.aamc.org/services/admissions-lifecycle/competencies-entering-medical-students

6. Tervalon, M., and J. Murray-García. "Cultural Humility versus Cultural Competence: A Critical Distinction in Defining Physician Training Outcomes in Multicultural Education." *J Health Care Poor U* 9, no. 2 (1998): 117–125. https://doi.org/10.1353/hpu.2010.0233

7. Kumagai, A.K., and M.L. Lypson. "Beyond Cultural Competence: Critical Consciousness, Social Justice, and Multicultural Education." *Acad Med* 84, no. 6 (2009): 782–787. https://doi.org/10.1097/ACM.0b013e3181a42398

8. Freire, P. *Education for Critical Consciousness.* New York: Continuum, 1993.

9. Wear, D., J. Zarconi, J.M. Aultman, M.R. Chyatte, and A.K. Kumagai. "Remembering Freddie Gray: Medical Education for Social Justice." *Acad Med* 92, no. 3 (2017): 312–17. https://doi.org/10.1097/ACM.0000000000001355

10. Campinha-Bacote, J. "Cultural Competemility: A Paradigm Shift in the Cultural Competence versus Cultural Humility Debate, Part I." *Online J Issues Nurs* 24, no. 1 (2019). https://doi.org/10.3912/OJIN.Vol24No01PPT20

11. World Health Organization. "About Social Determinants of Health." 2020. http://www.who.int/social_determinants/sdh_definition/en/.

12. Dahlgren, G., and M. Whitehead, M. "Policies and Strategies to Promote Social Equity in Health." Arbetsrapport 2007:14. Institute for Futures Studies, 1991.

13. U.S. Census Bureau. "QuickFacts: United States." 2019. https://www.census.gov/quickfacts/fact/table/US/PST045219

14. Centers for Disease Control and Prevention, "Disability Impacts All of Us Infographic." 2019. https://www.cdc.gov/ncbddd/disabilityandhealth/infographic-disability-impacts-all.html

15. University of Michigan, Center for Sustainable Systems. "U.S. Cities Factsheet." Pub. No. CSS09-06. 2020. http://css.umich.edu/factsheets/us-cities-factsheet

16. UCLA School of Law, Williams Institute. "LGBT Data & Demographics." 2019. https://williamsinstitute.law.ucla.edu/visualization/lgbt-stats/?topic=LGBT&so rtBy=percentage&sortDirection=descending#ranking

17. Centers for Disease Control and Prevention. "Disparities: Adolescent and School Health. 2018. https://www.cdc.gov/healthyyouth/disparities/index.htm

18. Sohn, H. "Racial and Ethnic Disparities in Health Insurance Coverage: Dynamics of Gaining and Losing Coverage over the Life-Course." *Popul Res Policy Rev* 36, no. 2 (2017): 181–201. https://doi.org/10.1007/s11113-016-9416-y

19. Centers for Disease Control and Prevention. "Coronavirus Disease 2019 (COVID-19)." 2020. https://www.cdc.gov/coronavirus/2019-ncov/need-extra-precautions/racial-ethnic-minorities.html

20. Ubhayakar, S., M. Capeless, R. Owens, K. Snorrason, and D. Zuckerman. "Anchor Mission Playbook." *Rush University Medical Center*. June 2017. https:// www.rush.edu/sites/default/files/anchor-mission-playbook.pdf.

21. Secretary's Advisory Committee on Health Promotion and Disease Prevention Objectives for 2020. "Healthy People 2020: An Opportunity to Address the Societal Determinants of Health in the United States." U.S. Department of Health and Human Services. July 26, 2010. http://www.healthypeople.gov/2010/ hp2020/advisory/SocietalDeterminantsHealth.htm.

22. Association of American Medical Colleges. "Diversity in Medicine: Facts and Figures 2019." 2019. https://www.aamc.org/data-reports/workforce/report/ diversity-medicine-facts-and-figures-2019

23. Harley, E.H. "The Forgotten History of Defunct Black Medical Schools in the 19th and 20th Centuries and the Impact of the Flexner Report." *J Natl Med Assoc* 98, no. 9 (2006): 1425–1429.

24. Hlavinka, E. "Racial Bias in Flexner Report Permeates Medical Education Today." *Medpage Today*. June 18, 2020. https://www.medpagetoday.com/ publichealthpolicy/medicaleducation/87171

25. Green, A.R., D.R. Carney, D.J. Pallin, L.H. Ngo, K.L. Raymond, L.I. Iezzoni, and M.R. Banaji. "Implicit Bias among Physicians and Its Prediction of Thrombolysis Decisions for Black and White Patients." *J Gen Intern Med* 22, no. 9 (2007): 1231–1238. https://doi.org/10.1007/s11606-007-0258-5

26. U.S. Department of Health and Human Services, Office of Minority Health, National Standards for Culturally and Linguistically Appropriate Services in Health and Health Care: Compendium of State-Sponsored National CLAS Standards Implementation Activities. Washington, DC: U.S. Department of Health and Human Services, 2016.

27. McGoldrick, M., J. Giordano, and N.G. Preto. *Ethnicity and Family Therapy*. 3rd ed. New York: Guilford Press, 2005.

28. Batalova, J., and J. Jie. "Language Diversity and English Proficiency in the United States in 2015." *Migrationpolicy*. November 11, 2016. https://www.migrationpolicy. org/article/language-diversity-and-english-proficiency-united-states-2015

29. Wilson, A., D. Martins-Welch, M. Williams, L. Tortez, A. Kozikowski, B. Earle, L. Attivissimo, L. Rosen, and R. Pekmezaris. "Risk Factor Assessment of Hospice Patients Readmitted within 7 Days of Acute Care Hospital Discharge." *Geriatrics* 3, no. 1 (2018): 4. https://doi.org/10.3390/geriatrics3010004

30. Divi, C., R.G. Koss, S.P. Schmaltz, and J.M. Loeb. "Language Proficiency and Adverse Events in US Hospitals: A Pilot Study." *Int J Qual Health C* 19, no. 2 (2007): 60–67. https://doi.org/10.1093/intqhc/mzl069

8

Teams in Medicine

For hundreds of years, medicine was not at its core a team-based profession. Each local community had one "all-knowing" doctor who would visit patients in their homes and treat whatever ailment they were suffering from, whether it be a mental disorder or an infection, using treatment modalities often grounded in both religious and scientific knowledge. But as modern healthcare has rapidly advanced, it has become exceedingly difficult for a single physician to possess the knowledge and skills necessary to treat all patients. The U.S. National Guideline Clearinghouse now lists over 2,700 clinical practice guidelines, and each year, the results of more than 25,000 new clinical trials are published.[1] No single person can absorb or use all of this information, and specialization and division of labor have become necessary. As the pace of innovation in healthcare continues to pick up, further advances in teamwork and division of labor are needed.

Even as the necessity of teams in medicine has been recognized, we have continued to educate our healthcare workforce in silos. We have hundreds of medical schools, thousands of nursing schools, and countless other health professional schools, and although they each educate professionals who will need to work in interprofessional teams, they may not be providing the knowledge and skills to do so. Because a large fraction of medical errors can be attributed to breakdowns in team skills, building effective teams has become a focus among medical educators. Interprofessional education (IPE) has been a step in the right direction, but current efforts are likely not enough. Medical education has changed over the years to reflect the increasing scientific knowledge base. Is it now time to modify its current paradigms to reflect the changing dynamics of healthcare delivery?

Task shifting and the paradigms of healthcare delivery

To improve access to medical care, particularly in the context of global health, a concept called "task-shifting" has gained favor. Task-shifting involves delegating certain responsibilities typically performed by physicians to other health professionals, such as nurses, physician assistants, and pharmacists. Research suggests that in low- and middle-income countries, task-shifting can save costs and improve efficiency, ultimately improving population health.[2] Furthermore, what is colloquially referred to as "medical deserts" exist in the United States, where there is little or no access to physicians; task-shifting of physician responsibilities to other professional healthcare providers has been suggested to improve access to care in these areas. Some policymakers also have focused on creating initiatives for recruiting physicians to underserved areas, such as through the establishment of medical schools in these regions and through financial incentives for physicians practicing in rural areas.[3]

Currently, an estimated 30 million Americans reside over 60 minutes away from a hospital that provides trauma care, and the federal government has classified nearly 80 percent of the rural population of the United States as medically underserved.[4] Additionally, approximately 20 percent of Americans live in rural regions, but only 9 percent of the country's doctors practice in rural areas, and this situation is predicted to only get worse.[5] To address these issues of access to care, the United States has begun to mirror global health initiatives of task-shifting responsibilities to nurses, physician assistants, and pharmacists in providing care.

While preliminary studies suggest that these nonphysician providers are effective in their new roles in primary care teams,[6] these initiatives have largely been met with questions by physicians. Will physician authority be diminished? Are providers with less experience or less education not properly qualified to perform these kinds of tasks? Some may view task shifting as part of a McDonaldization of medicine, in which important values such as care for the individual and the sanctity of the patient–physician relationship are threatened to improve efficiency, calculability, predictability, and control in medicine.[7]

Improving access to care is sure to require a multipronged approach. An interdisciplinary approach to healthcare, involving integration of knowledge and sharing of responsibilities among physicians and other members of the healthcare team, is likely to be a part of the solution. However, although we are striving for interdisciplinary teams in healthcare, we have continued to educate our future healthcare workforce in silos. Even when we form healthcare teams with members of different healthcare professions, they are often multidisciplinary rather than interdisciplinary (see Table 8.1).[8]

Integration of knowledge and skills from multiple professions is a goal of an interdisciplinary team. However, limited structured opportunities exist in medical school or residency curricula for physicians to learn how to evaluate the knowledge and competencies of nonphysician providers, and vice versa. There are significant obstacles to cohesive interdisciplinary teamwork, because each profession possesses a unique culture with a specific set of values, approaches, and behaviors that develop through education and socialization. Accordingly, there is a need for formal interdisciplinary training.

In this chapter, we first describe the historical perspective of teams in medicine, especially as it regards to changes in hierarchy, and suggest that medicine will continue to evolve, particularly in paradigms of healthcare delivery. However, we also suggest that these changes ought not to cause physicians undue worry. Although the physician's role will continue to change, as medical professionals we have a responsibility to ourselves and our profession to put ourselves in a position to adapt. As discussed in Chapter 3 of this volume, adapting to the changing roles of physicians in healthcare may be best served through a lens of expectation management, while keeping happiness as a goal.

Table 8.1 Multidisciplinary versus Interdisciplinary Teams

Multidisciplinary Teams	Interdisciplinary Teams
Involve team members from different professions who work independently of each other to deliver care	Involve team members from different professions who collaborate with each other to deliver care
Additive knowledge of members	Synergistic knowledge of members
Share information on a minimal basis	Share information continually and integrate into solutions
Members of the team function in their areas of expertise	Members of the team function in their areas of expertise

Historical perspectives of teams in medicine

Formal initiatives for teamwork in medicine have only existed for the past hundred years or so. Literature on the topic dates only as far back as the early 20th century, when Richard Cabot at Massachusetts General Hospital wrote in support of doctors, educators, and social workers working together as a team.[9] Incorporation of teamwork in practice was first pioneered at the Mayo Clinic before World War I, and in the United Kingdom by Alfred Keogh, the wartime director-general of the army medical service, who referred to "surgical firms" and "surgical teams" interchangeably.[10] World War II also showcased the benefits of approaching healthcare with multidisciplinary teams. As a result of the war, the fields of surgery, burns, rehabilitation, cleft palate, long-term care, and mental health became distinctly team-based.[11]

Medical education began to reflect changing opinions about the need for teams in medicine in the 1960s. This wave was stimulated by President Johnson's program for the Great Society and the War on Poverty, which focused on providing more efficient primary healthcare and facilitating cooperation between internists, pediatricians, nurses, and family health workers. The concept of interdisciplinary teams of health professionals was seen as a means for providing comprehensive and continuous care to poor and underserved populations. Students in the health professions began to seek out interdisciplinary projects, particularly in the summer months. Interest has been sustained since that time, and IPE initiatives have gained traction as ways for healthcare professionals to collaborate and learn from one another.

A further push toward team-based healthcare gained traction with the publication of the National Academy of Medicine's report *To Err Is Human*, which identified high rates of medical errors, many of which were suggested to stem from dysfunctional teamwork.[12] Teamwork began to be viewed as necessary for ensuring patient safety. More recently, provisions in the Patient Protection and Affordable Care Act and by the World Health Organization serve as mandates for teamwork in medicine. According to the World Health Organization, "it is no longer enough for health workers to be professional. In the current global climate, health workers also need to be interprofessional."[13]

However, one of the challenges faced in bringing different healthcare professions together is that, unless trained to do so, professionals may have difficulty working together in a truly integrated way. Despite the increased prevalence of team-based care, The Joint Commission found that the root cause of 68.3 percent of preventable sentinel events involved breakdown of teamwork factors, including communication (discussed in further detail in Chapter 6 of this volume).[14] The Interprofessional Education Collaborative was established in 2009 to address this concern and in 2011 published educational competencies to support healthcare curricula move toward better integration of this approach in their training.[15]

The healthcare team has historically been constructed in a hierarchical manner, because an effective team requires strong leadership to promote coordination and communication. A social hierarchy, where medical doctors are positioned at the top, has long existed and remained even as other health professions gain responsibility and autonomy. When considering the hierarchy of medical teams, the historical relationship between the physician and nurse is important to consider. Although many other health professions exist and are undeniably important, nurses and physicians have long been the two largest professional groups in healthcare and are thus central to interprofessional, collaborative care. Althought the relationship between physicians and nurses has changed overtime it is fundamentally rooted in mutual respect and interprofessional collaboration.[16]

The process of professional socialization occurs in differential ways within the health professions and influences dynamics within healthcare teams. Early preprofessional socialization has been shown to significantly impact practicing physicians' perceptions, expectations, and practices.[17] By better understanding the sociohistorical contexts behind how these roles are perceived, we can better promote respect and collaboration as well as gain better insight into the realities of each of the healthcare professions.

Historically, the physician–nurse relationship was not only hierarchical but also patriarchal.[18] Role differences between nurses and doctors have been interpreted to mirror the gender division of labor in everyday life, with nurses maintaining the nurturing environment while working at the bedside and doctors making the impactful, core decisions of medicine.[19] However, just as gender divisions in medicine continue to evolve—indeed, women only were able to join the physician workforce beginning in the 1970s, but now compose over a third of the workforce and half of residents in training and medical school classes in the United States[20]—the hierarchically and patriarchally shaped roles of the physician and nurse are changing as well.

The roles of other members of the healthcare team also are evolving. Reflecting a demand for primary care providers, nurse practitioners (NPs) and physician assistants (PAs) are beginning to play increased roles in diagnostics and patient evaluations.[21] In some states, NPs and PAs have prescribing authority and are able to provide primary care without a physician present. While it may, at first, seem that physicians have reduced responsibility and autonomy, these changes to the paradigms of healthcare delivery may actually benefit physicians by freeing up time and mental bandwidth to focus on more specialized responsibilities, reducing their clerical and administrative burden.[22] Furthermore, as artificial intelligence begins to play a larger role in healthcare, it may potentially play a helpful role as a "member" of the healthcare team (see Chapter 4 of this volume).[23] These changes may work to promote professional well-being and protect against physician burnout.

Effective teams in medicine

What, exactly, is a team, and what does teamwork look like in medicine? Academic research on teams has consistently grown over the past 30 or so years, and as a result, many definitions have been developed. In general, a team consists of two or more individuals with defined roles who coordinate to perform specific tasks to realize a shared goal or outcome.[24] Salas and colleagues suggest that effective teams consist of individuals who possess the knowledge, skills, and attitudes (KSAs) necessary for effective teamwork.[25] These KSAs include characteristics such as assertiveness and mutual trust. Mutual trust involves a shared belief that team members will protect and support the interests of their team.[26] Team members with mutual trust are willing to admit to mistakes and accept and appreciate feedback.[27] This allows them to firmly assert their concerns even to a higher-ranking team member without fear of reprisal. Other teamwork KSAs include team leadership, mutual performance monitoring, and adaptability (see Table 8.2). Teamwork in medicine depends on each team member being able to anticipate the needs of others, adjust to each other's actions, and possess a shared understanding of how a procedure should happen.

Table 8.2 Team Knowledge, Skills, and Attitudes (KSAs) Competencies and Outcomes

Teamwork	Definition	Behavioral Examples
Team leadership	Ability to direct and coordinate the activities of other team members, assess team performance, assign tasks, develop team KSAs, motivate team members, plan and organize, and establish a positive atmosphere	Facilitate team problem Provide performance expectations and acceptable interaction patterns. synchronize and combine individual team member contributions Seek and evaluate information that impacts team functioning Clarify team member roles Engage In preparatory meetings and feedback sessions with the team
Mutual performance monitoring (aka situation monitoring)	The ability to develop common understandings of the team environment and apply appropriate task strategies in order to accurately monitor teammate performance	Identifying mistakes and laps in other team members actions Providing feedback regarding team member actions In order to facilitate self-correction
Backup behavior (aka mutual support)	Ability to anticipate other team member's needs through accurate knowledge about their responsibilities The ability to shift workload among members to achieve balance during high periods of workloads or pressure	Recognition by potential backup providers that there is a workload distribution problem in their team Shifting of work responsibilities to under-utilized team members Completion of the whole task or parts o0f tasks by other team member
Adaptability	Ability to adjust strategies based on information gathered from the environment through the use of compensatory behavior and reallocation of intra team resources. Although a course of action or team report ire in response to changing condition(internal or external)	Identify cues that a change has occurred, assign meaning to that change, and develop a new plan to deal with the changes Identify opportunities for improvement and innovation for habitual routine practices Remain vigilant to changes in the internal and external environment the team

Adapted from D.P. Baker, R. Day, and E. Salas, "Teamwork as an Essential Component of High-Reliability Organizations," *Health Serv Res* 41(4 Pt 2) (2006): 1581-82, https://doi.org/10.1111/j.1475-6773.2006.00566.x.

Types of healthcare teams in medicine

Teams in medicine may have different purposes: consider office-based teams, disaster response teams, hospice teams, or emergency room teams that care for acutely ill patients, among many others. Teams may also differ in composition and modality of collaboration. In a study of primary care teams, Saint-Pierre and colleagues found that they could be appropriately grouped into four types by composition:

1. Specialized teams, consisting of one primary care doctor and one specialist, who interact with one or more professionals from other primary care disciplines.
2. Highly multidisciplinary teams, which consist of a doctor–nurse duo that work with the support of a nutritionist or other specialist, as well as with the participation of at least one professional from a complementary discipline, such as a podiatrist, midwife, or counselor.
3. Doctor–nurse–pharmacist team, who function with the support of other primary-care professionals.
4. Physician–nurse–centered teams, who function with the support of other primary care professionals.[28]

Furthermore, the authors identified four categories of primary care teams classified by type of collaboration:

1. Co-located collaboration, in which team members work in a highly coordinated manner through regular meetings and direct communication, but without shared consultations.
2. Nonhierarchical collaboration, in which teams do not have a clinical leader.
3. Collaboration through shared consultations.
4. Collaboration via referral and counterreferral, which is not necessarily interdisciplinary.

It is evident that there are many different types of teams in medicine, especially when we consider that these authors' classifications of teams were in primary care alone.

The diversity of teams in medicine creates challenges in defining guidelines for optimal teamwork. However, core principles that are consistently demonstrated by effective teams have been identified. In Box 8.1, the five core competencies of healthcare teams suggested by the National Academy of Medicine are described.[29]

Box 8.1 **Five Core Competencies of Healthcare Teams**

1. *Provide patient-centered care*: Identify, respect, and care about patients' differences, values, preferences, and expressed needs; relieve pain and suffering; coordinate continuous care; listen to, clearly inform, communicate with, and educate patients; share decision-making and management; and continuously advocate disease prevention, wellness, and promotion of healthy lifestyles, including a focus on population health.
2. *Work in interdisciplinary teams*: Cooperate, collaborate, communicate, and integrate care in teams to ensure that care is continuous and reliable.
3. *Employ evidence-based practice*: Integrate best research with clinical expertise and patient values for optimum care and participate in learning and research activities to the extent feasible.
4. *Apply quality improvement*: Identify errors and hazards in care; understand and implement basic safety-design principles, such as standardization and simplification; continually understand and measure quality of care in terms of structure, process, and outcomes in relation to patient and community needs; design and test interventions to change processes and systems of care, with the objective of improving quality.
5. *Utilize informatics*: Communicate, manage knowledge, mitigate error, and support decision-making using information technology.

Adapted from A.C. Greiner and E. Knebel, eds., *Health Professions Education: A Bridge to Quality* (Washington, DC: National Academies Press, 2003), Figure 3.1, https://www.ncbi.nlm.nih.gov/books/NBK221519/.

Healthcare teams have historically had a physician at the head. Another way to promote diversity in healthcare is the formation of some teams with a less-structured hierarchy, or with NPs or PAs at the head. In many states, collaboration agreements must be in place with physicians, while in other states, healthcare teams may not require a physician. In many situations, physicians may not be present while care is provided by nonphysician team members but may still be liable and exposed to malpractice risk. Legal issues surrounding the evolving medical team are likely to remain unresolved until widespread adoption and subsequent litigation occurs, but it is important for physicians to be aware of the potential for novel ethical and legal issues regarding teams in medicine. (The physician's role as an employee is further discussed in Chapter 16 of this volume.)

Benefits of effective teamwork among diverse team settings

The importance of teamwork has been heavily researched in medicine and other disciplines that work in critical and high-intensity environments. Medicine is an example of a high reliability organization (HRO), is which the consequences of errors are high but the incidence of errors is low. While conclusive evidence that effective teamwork leads to increased health outcomes has not yet been established, it has been shown to lead to increased outcomes in other HROs,[30] suggesting that healthcare outcomes should be positively affected by teamwork as well.

The concept of "collective intelligence" states that the most effective teams are not the ones with the most intelligent or capable individuals, but rather the teams that include multiple perspectives in making their decisions and have members who are socially perceptive.[31] For a team to function effectively, members of the team should possess diverse perspectives and be comfortable sharing relevant knowledge with other members of the team, a concept referred to as "expertise use." However, expertise use requires an environment of psychological safety, which refers to "a sense of confidence that the team will not embarrass, reject, or punish someone for speaking up."[32p354]

Evidence also suggests that effective team environments can promote psychological well-being and protect against burnout. Dysfunctional teamwork has been cited as a predictor for decreased well-being of healthcare providers[33] and increased acute and chronic clinician strain in nurses.[34] On the other hand, strong team culture may protect against exhaustion and disengagement in the healthcare team. Positive perceptions toward teamwork was associated with better mental health in physicians.[35] Furthermore, a study suggests that strong team culture and team structures that promote strong team culture are associated with lower burnout in primary care.[36] An initiative of The National Academy of Medicine to combat burnout includes reorganizing work so that tasks are more optimally distributed. [37]

The resilience activation framework was developed to explain how access to social resources leads to adaptation and recovery in postdisaster settings. We believe that it also provides an appropriate model for teamwork that leads to resilience against physician burnout. According to this framework, most people are inherently resilient, but "exposure to harm leads to resource loss, stress, and psychological reactivity." However, "access to or engagement with community/social resources can activate inherent individual resilience attributes."[38p49] Along these lines, we believe that physicians are inherently resilient but are currently suffering due to unprecedented systemic issues (see Chapter 10 of this volume). However, by building a community of practice that is healthy, engaging, and socially supportive, physicians may be more equipped to develop resilience. Resilience has been suggested to consist of two components: *activation* and *decompression*.[39] The concept of activation represents the ability to be engaged with work and to interpret one's work as effective and meaningful. Decompression represents the ability to separate oneself from work and experience a healthy mindset when one is not at work. Effective teamwork can help to improve both activation and decompression.

The shift from individual medical practitioners to interdependent health teams has increased physician's reliance on other physicians and healthcare professionals. In modern hospitals and practices, there are varying, diverse teams for purposes such as rapid response, surgery, palliative care, and specific disease treatment. Overall, for the benefit of patients and physicians themselves, utilizing the skills underlying effective teamwork is important for all healthcare professionals.

Educational and other initiatives to develop teamwork skills

The importance of teamwork can be seen in the incorporation and expansion of education focused on teamwork skills in both medical student education and continuing medical education for practicing physicians. Specific, targeted training to improve teamwork is critical as research has shown that teamwork issues play an important role in causing preventable medical errors that may lead to adverse events for patients. For example, in surgery—a highly coordinated process between many surgical team members—teamwork and communication problems are the strongest predictors of the frequency of surgical errors. However, effective teamwork with constant communication, mutual respect, and strength of respect was associated with less minor negative problems, shorter operating times, and decreased hospital stays.[40]

In practice, healthcare teams are comprised of a diverse set of healthcare professionals, including physicians, nurses, allied health professionals, medical technicians, and social workers. This creates a need to balance the roles to prevent an unequal distribution of duties or issues associated with *role blurring* while maintaining shared goals and problem-solving.[41] To overcome this barrier, there have been recent efforts to implement IPE. IPE involves different health professionals participating in interactive learning activities together. Preliminary evidence has shown that IPE leads to improved patient satisfaction, collaborative team behavior, and reduced clinical errors.[42]

Borrowing from other high-reliability organizations, healthcare team training was originally modeled on crew resource management (CRM), a concept developed for training in aviation. CRM focuses on a specific set of team competencies, including hazard identification, assertive communication, and collective management of resources.[43] However, team training in medicine now encompasses a much broader understanding of teams. Many team-training tools currently exist in practice to help medical professionals continue to develop and maintain values and skills to support their teamwork. Team-training initiatives have been adopted across a wide range of acute care settings, including academic hospitals[44] and community-based hospitals, [45] as well as medical centers affiliated with the Veterans Administration[46,] and the Military Health System.[47]

One of the best-known and most highly adopted programs, TeamSTEPPS, was developed collaboratively by the Agency for Healthcare Research and Quality and the Department of Defense and first implemented in 2006.[48] It aims to develop team skills, including leadership, situation monitoring, mutual support, and communication.[48] The group developed the situation, background, assessment, and recommendation model of communication to help further its goals. Furthermore, practical case studies and video vignettes were created to reinforce learning. The TeamSTEPPS initiative also includes an implementation and sustainment plan to facilitate organizational change.

Simulation-based training is a common modality for learning teamwork. Through this training, students are immersed in experiential learning situations that simulate real-world scenarios where they can directly apply skills. Examples of these exercises include scenarios revolving around crisis situations, critical decision-making moments, or role play with patients.[49] Technology has facilitated simulation-based learning in high-fidelity patient simulations that utilize computerized mannequins to provide realistic examples of procedures or situations for student practice. Reviews of high-fidelity patient simulations show that essential components for educational learning include educational feedback, repetitive practice, and ranges of difficulty and clinical conditions.[50]

In addition to formal team training, many medical schools have implemented pedagogical methods that heavily emphasize teamwork, notably team-based learning (TBL) and problem-based learning (PBL). TBL is an instructional technique originally implemented in business schools and is designed to develop high-performing teams and engage students in active learning.[51] The core scheduled components of TBL sessions include

1. Advanced preparation assignment before the in-person learning.
2. Individual and group readiness tests to evaluate understanding of content.
3. Group application activity to use material from the preparation assignment in a real-world scenario.

The groups are usually created in sizes of five to six students, which are smaller than PBL groups.

PBL is an educational approach that involves working in groups to solve open-ended problems. Although mixed results are often reported regarding the efficacy of TBL and PBL, most studies show that although there are not proven large increases in exam scores, there are improvements in peer inter-actions, active learning, and student participation.[52] Some studies suggest that a hybrid approach that combines the strength of TBL and PBL instruc-tional design will improve outcomes for learners. The pedagogical modal-ities of TBL and PBL are described in Table 8.3.

The strengths of TBL include creating heterogeneous teams of varying skill sets, stressing accountability, providing real-world scenarios, and pro-viding student feedback.[53] Further research on the effectiveness of TBL and PBL is still being conducted. However, the positive student perceptions of

Table 8.3 The Major Differences between Team-Based Learning and Problem-Based Learning Sessions

	Team-Based Learning	Problem-Based Learning
Group size	5–6 students	6–10 students
Group assignments	Purposefully assigned with varying skill sets	Random assignment
Time spent in groups	An entire course	6–10 weeks then rotations
Instructors	One teacher oversees multiple teams	One teacher assigned to each group
Assignments	Individual assignments completed before sharing and discussion in groups; no preclass assignments	Assignments before group work in class, individual, and group-consensus tests
Physical location of groups	In separate rooms	In same large room
Content generation	Students generate topics to study and identify unknown information	Teacher creates content based on specific knowledge to apply to situations
Peer feedback	No peer evaluations	Peer evaluations and feedback

Adapted from D. Dolmans, L. Michaelsen, J. van Merriënboer, and C. van der Vleuten, "Should We Choose between Problem-Based Learning and Team-Based Learning? No, Combine the Best of Both Worlds!" *Med Teach* 37, no. 4 (2015): 354–359, https://doi.org/10.3109/0142159X.2014.948828, reprinted by permission of the publisher (Taylor & Francis Ltd, http://www.tandfonline.com).

instructional models that involve teamwork and provide for active student engagement allow for effective incorporation of team learning in medical education compared to lecture settings.

Chapter Quick Summary

- Healthcare continues to become more team-based, but we continue to educate our healthcare providers in silos.
- Interprofessional education (IPE) is a step in the right direction for developing effective healthcare teams.
- The trend toward task-shifting means that there are now healthcare teams that do not have a physician at the head.
- Effective teams consist of members who possess teamwork knowledge, skills, and attitudes (KSAs). These include assertiveness, mutual trust, team leadership, mutual performance monitoring, and adaptability.
- Medicine is an example of a high-reliability organization (HRO), in which the consequences of errors are high, but the incidence of errors is low. Teamwork has been shown to be particularly important for HROs.
- Teamwork can be learned through IPE, including programs derived from Crew Resource Management and TeamSTEPPS.
- Simulation-based training, as well as team-based learning and problem-based learning, may also be effective modalities for learning teamwork.

Resources

American Medical Association. "What Makes Team-Based Care Effective?" [CME course]. November 14, 2019. https://edhub.ama-assn.org/health-systems-science/interactive/18028227

MedEd Portal Interprofessional Education. [Home page]. https://www.mededportal.org/interprofessional-education

Mitchell, P., M. Wynia, R. Golden, B. McNellis, S. Okun, C.E. Webb, V. Rohrbach, and I. Von Kohorn. "Core Principles & Values of Effective Team-Based Health

Care." Discussion Paper, Institute of Medicine. October 2012. https://nam.edu/wp-content/uploads/2015/06/VSRT-Team-Based-Care-Principles-Values.pdf

World Health Organization. "WHO Safety Curriculum Topic 4: Being an Effective Team Player." https://www.who.int/patientsafety/education/curriculum/who_mc_topic-4.pdf

References

1. Mancher, M., D.M. Wolman, S. Greenfield, and E. Steinberg, eds. *Clinical Practice Guidelines We Can Trust.* Washington, DC: National Academies Press, 2001.
2. Seidman, G., and R. Atun. "Does Task Shifting Yield Cost Savings and Improve Efficiency for Health Systems? A Systematic Review of Evidence from Low-Income and Middle-income Countrie." *Hum Res Health* 15, no. 1 (2017): 29. https://doi.org/10.1186/s12960-017-0200-9
3. Jutzi, L., K. Vogt, E. Drever, and J. Nisker. "Recruiting Medical Students to Rural Practice." *Can Fam Physician* 55, no. 1 (2009): 72–73.
4. Agency for Health care Research and Quality. "National Health Care Quality and Disparities Report: Chartbook on Rural Health Care." AHRQ Pub. No. 17(18)-0001-2-EF. October 2017. https://www.ahrq.gov/research/findings/nhqrdr/chartbooks/ruralhealth/index.html
5. Rosenblatt, R.A., and L.G. Hart. "Physicians and Rural America." *Western J Med* 173, no. 5 (2000): 348–351.
6. Everett, C.M., C.T. Thorpe, M. Palta, P. Carayon, C. Bartels, and M.A. Smith. "Physician Assistants and Nurse Practitioners Perform Effective Roles on Teams Caring for Medicare Patients with Diabetes." *Health Affair (Project Hope)* 32, no. 11 (2013): 1942–1948. https://doi.org/10.1377/hlthaff.2013.0506
7. Dorsey, E.R., and G. Ritzer. "The McDonaldization of Medicine." *JAMA Neurol* 73, no. 1 (2016): 15–16. https://doi.org/10.1001/jamaneurol.2015.3449
8. Jessup, R.L. "Interdisciplinary versus Multidisciplinary Care Teams: Do We Understand the Difference?" *Aust Health Rev* 31, no. 3 (2007): 330.
9. Cabot, R.C. *Social Service and the Art of Healing.* New York: Moffat, Yard, 1909.
10. Cooter, R. "Keywords in the History of Medicine Teamwork." *Lancet* 363, no. 9416 (2004): 1245. https://doi.org/10.1016/S0140-6736(04)15977-1
11. Baldwin, D.C., Jr. "Some Historical Notes on Interdisciplinary and Interprofessional Education and Practice in Health Care in the USA." *J Interprof Care* 21, Supp.1 (2007): 23–37. https://doi.org/10.1080/13561820701594728

12. Kohn, L.T., J.M. Corrigan, & M.S. Donaldson, eds. To Err is Human: Building a Safer Health System. Washington, DC: National Academies Press, 2000.

13. World Health Organization. "Framework for Action on Interprofessional Education and Collaborative Practice." 2010. http://whqlibdoc.who.int/hq/2010/WHO_HRH_HPN_10.3_eng.pdf

14. Joint Commission. Root Cause Analysis in Health Care: A Joint Commission Guide to Analysis and Corrective Action of Sentinel and Adverse Events. 7th ed. Oakbridge Terrace, IL: Joint Commission, 2020.

15. Schmitt, M., A. Blue, C.A. Aschenbrener, and T.R. Viggiano. "Core Competencies for Interprofessional Collaborative Practice: Reforming Health Care by Transforming Health Professionals' Education." Acad Med 86, no. 11 (2011): 1351. https://doi.org/10.1097/ACM.0b013e3182308e39

16. Price, S., S. Doucet, and L.M. Hall. "The Historical Social Positioning of Nursing and Medicine: Implications for Career Choice, Early Socialization and Interprofessional Collaboration." J Interprof Care 28, no. 2 (2014): 103–109. https://doi.org/10.3109/13561820.2013.867839

17. Day, R.A., P.A. Field, I.E. Campbell, and L. Reutter. "Students' Evolving Beliefs about Nursing: From Entry to Graduation in a Four-year Baccalaureate Programme." Nurs Educ Today 15, no. 5 (1995): 357–364.

18. Sweet, S.J., and I.J. Norman. "The Nurse–Doctor Relationship: A Selective Literature Review." J Adv Nurs 22, no. 1 (1995): 165–170. https://doi.org/10.1046/j.1365-2648.1995.22010165.x

19. Oakley, A. "What Price Professionalism? The Importance of Being a Nurse." Nurs Times 80, no. 50 (1984): 24–27.

20. American Association of Medical Colleges. "Diversity in Medicine: Facts and Figures 2019." 2019. https://www.aamc.org/data-reports/workforce/report/diversity-medicine-facts-and-figures-2019

21. Everett, C.M., J.R. Schumacher, A. Wright, and M.A. Smith. "Physician Assistants and Nurse Practitioners as a Usual Source of Care." J Rural Health 25, no. 4 (2009): 407–414. https://doi.org/10.1111/j.1748-0361.2009.00252.x

22. Bakanas, E.L. "Resistance to Changing Roles in the Medical Team." AMA J Ethics 13, no. 6 (2013): 498–503. https://doi.org/10.1001/virtualmentor.2013.15.6.ecas2-1306

23. Ieva, A.D. "AI-Augmented Multidisciplinary Teams: Hype or Hope?" Lancet 394, no. 10211 (2019): 1801. https://doi.org/10.1016/S0140-6736(19)32626-1

24. Salas, E., and J.A. Cannon-Bowers. "The Science of Training: A Decade of Progress." Annu Rev Psychol 52 (2001): 471–499. https://doi.org/10.1146/annurev.psych.52.1.471

25. Baker, D.P., R. Day, and E. Salas. "Teamwork as an Essential Component of High-Reliability Organizations." *Health Serv Res* 41, no. 4, pt. 2 (2016): 1576–1598. https://doi.org/10.1111/j.1475-6773.2006.00566.x

26. Salas, E., D.E. Sims, and C.S. Burke. "Is There a 'Big Five' in Teamwork?" *Small Group Res* 36, no. 5 (2005): 555–599. https://doi.org/10.1177/1046496405277134

27. Bandow, D. "Time to Create Sound Teamwork." *J Qual Part* 24 (2001): 41–47.

28. Saint-Pierre, C., V. Herskovic, and M. Sepúlveda. "Multidisciplinary Collaboration in Primary Care: A Systematic Review." *Fam Pract* 35, no. 2 (2018): 132–141. https://doi.org/10.1093/fampra/cmx085

29. Greiner, A.C., and E. Knebel, eds. *Health Professions Education: A Bridge to Quality.* Washington, DC: National Academies Press, 2003.

30. Salas, E., C.A. Bowers, and J.A. Cannon-Bowers. "Military Team Research: 10 Years of Progress." *Milit Psychol* 7, no. 2 (1995): 55–75.

31. Woolley, A.W., I. Aggarwal, I., and T.W. Malone. "Collective Intelligence and Group Performance." *Curr Dir Psychol Sci* 24, no. 6 (2015): 420–424. https://doi.org/10.1177/0963721415599543

32. Edmondson, A. "Psychological Safety and Learning Behavior in Work Teams." *Admin Sci Quart* 44, no. 2 (1999): 350–383. https://doi.org/10.2307/2666999

33. Merlani, P., M. Verdon, A. Businger, G. Domenighetti, H. Pargger, and B. Ricou. "Burnout in ICU Caregivers: A Multicenter Study of Factors Associated to Centers." *Am J Resp Crit Care* 184, no. 10 (2011): 1140–1146. https://doi.org/10.1164/rccm.201101-0068OC

34. Gabriel, A.S., J.M. Diefendorff, and R.J. Erickson. "The Relations of Daily Task Accomplishment Satisfaction with Changes in Affect: A Multilevel Study in Nurses." *J Appl Psychol* 96, no. 5 (2011): 1095–1104. https://doi.org/10.1037/a0023937

35. Sutinen, R., M. Kivimäki, M. Elovainio, and P. Forma. "Associations between Stress at Work and Attitudes towards Retirement in Hospital Physicians." *Work Stress* 19, no. 2 (2005): 177–185. https://doi.org/10.1080/02678370500151760

36. Willard-Grace, R., D. Hessler, E. Rogers, K. Dubé, T. Bodenheimer, and K. Grumbach. "Team Structure and Culture Are Associated with Lower Burnout in Primary Care." *JABFM* 27, no. 2 (2014): 229–238. https://doi.org/10.3122/jabfm.2014.02.130215

37. National Academies of Sciences, Engineering, and Medicine; National Academy of Medicine; and Committee on Systems Approaches to Improve Patient Care by Supporting Clinician Well-Being. *Taking Action Against Clinician Burnout: A*

Systems Approach to Professional Well-Being. Washington, DC: National Academies Press, 2019.

38. Abramson, D.M., L.M. Grattan, B. Mayer, C.E. Colten, F.A. Arosemena, A. Rung, and M. Lichtveld. "The Resilience Activation Framework: A Conceptual Model of How Access to Social Resources Promotes Adaptation and Rapid Recovery in Post-disaster Settings." *J Behav Health Serv R* 42, no. 1 (2015): 42–57. https://doi. org/10.1007/s11414-014-9410-2

39. Howell, T.G., D.E. Mylod, T.H. Lee, T. Shanafelt, and P. Prissel. "Physician Burnout, Resilience, and Patient Experience in a Community Practice: Correlations and the Central Role of Activation." *J Patient Exper* (2019): 1–10. https://doi.org/ 10.1177/2374373519888343

40. Manser, T. "Teamwork and Patient Safety in Dynamic Domains of Health Care: A Review of the Literature." *Acta Anaesth Scan* 53, no. 2 (2005): 143–151. https://doi.org/10.1111/j.1399-6576.2008.01717.x

41. Hall, P. "Interprofessional Teamwork: Professional Cultures as Barriers." *J Interprof Care* 19 (2005): 188–196.

42. Reeves, S., M. Zwarenstein, J. Goldman, H. Barr, D. Freeth, M. Hammick, and I. Koppel. "Interprofessional Education: Effects on Professional Practice and Health Care Outcomes." *Cochrane DB Syst Rev* 1 (2008). https://doi.org/10.1002/ 14651858.CD002213.pub2

43. Salas, E., C.S. Burke, C.A. Bowers, and K.A. Wilson. "Team Training in the Skies: Does Crew Resource Management (CRM) Training Work?" *Hum Factors* 43, no. 4 (2001): 641–74. https://doi.org/10.1518/001872001775870386

44. Mayer, C.M., L. Cluff, W.-T. Lin, T.S. Willis, R.E. Stafford, C. Williams, R. Saunders, K.A. Short, N. Lenfestey, H.L. Kane, and J.B. Amoozegar. "Evaluating Efforts to Optimize TeamSTEPPS Implementation in Surgical and Pediatric Intensive Care Units." *Joint Comm J Qual Pat Safety* 37, no. 8 (2011): 365–374. https://doi.org/10.1016/s1553-7250(11)37047-x

45. Riley, W., S. Davis, K. Miller, H. Hansen, F. Sainfort, and R. Sweet. "Didactic and Simulation Nontechnical Skills Team Training to Improve Perinatal Patient Outcomes in a Community Hospital." *Joint Comm J Qual Pat Safety* 37, no. 8 (2011): 357–364. https://doi.org/10.1016/s1553-7250(11)37046-8

46. Neily, J., P.D. Mills, Y. Young-Xu, B.T. Carney, P. West, D.H. Berger, L.M. Mazzia, D.E. Paull, and J.P. Bagian. "Association between Implementation of a Medical Team Training Program and Surgical Mortality." *JAMA* 304, no. 15 (2010): 1693–1700. https://doi.org/10.1001/jama.2010.1506

47. Deering, S., M.A. Rosen, V. Ludi, M. Munroe, A. Pocrnich, C. Laky, and P.G. Napolitano. "On the Front Lines of Patient Safety: Implementation and Evaluation of Team Training in Iraq." *Joint Comm J Qual Pat Safety* 37, no. 8 (2011): 350–356. https://doi.org/10.1016/s1553-7250(11)37045-6

48. King, H.B., J. Battles, D.P. Baker, A. Alonso, E. Salas, J. Webster, L. Toomey, and M. Salisbury. "TeamSTEPPS®: Strategies and Tools to Enhance Performance and Patient Safety." In *Advances in Patient Safety: New Directions and Alternative Approaches*, Vol. 3: *Performance and Tools*. Edited by K. Henriksen, J.B. Battles, M.A. Keyes, and M.L. Grady. Falls Church, VA: Agency for Healthcare Research and Quality, 2008. https://www.ncbi.nlm.nih.gov/books/NBK43686

49. Banerjee, A., J.M. Slagle, N.D. Mercaldo, R. Booker, A. Miller, D.J. France, L. Rawn, and M.B. Weinger. "A Simulation-based Curriculum to Introduce Key Teamwork Principles to Entering Medical Students." *BMC Med Educ* 16, no. 1 (2016): 295. https://doi.org/10.1186/s12909-016-0808-9

50. Issenberg, S.B., W.C. Mcgaghie, E.R. Petrusa, D.L. Gordon, and R.J. Scalese. "Features and Uses of High-fidelity Medical Simulations that Lead to Effective Learning: A BEME Systematic Review." *Med Teach* 27, no. 1 (2005): 10–28. https://doi.org/10.1080/01421590500046924

51. Michaelsen, L., A. Knight, and L. Fink. *Team-Based Learning: A Transformative Use of Small Groups in College Teaching*. Sterling, VA: Stylus, 2004.

52. Reimschisel, T., A.L. Herring, J. Huang, and T.J. Minor. "A Systematic Review of the Published Literature on Team-based Learning in Health Professions Education." *Med Teach* 39, no. 12, (2017): 1227–1237. https://doi.org/10.1080/0142159X.2017.1340636

53. Sisk, R.J. "Team-Based Learning: Systematic Research Review." *J Nurs Educ* 50, no. 12 (2011): 665–669. https://doi.org/10.3928/01484834-20111017-01

9
Lifestyle Medicine

Physicians give plenty of general health advice to their patients and society at large. If we were to have our way, everyone would exercise, wash their hands often and get their flu shots, cover their mouths when they sneeze, avoid tobacco products, and use plenty of sunscreen every time they went outdoors. Indeed, the growing scientific and medical literature overwhelmingly supports the fact that daily habits and actions have serious consequences on health and quality of life. As medical professionals, we have a mandate to practice evidence-based medicine and promote the health of our patients. However, current efforts to stem the tide of chronic disease in the United States have been insufficient.

The impact of chronic diseases on health and quality of life are well-known among the medical community. The COVID-19 pandemic has also served as a wake-up call. People with underlying medical conditions have been shown to be at increased risk for severe illness from COVID-19; according to the initial findings by the Centers for Disease Control and Prevention (CDC), hospitalization rates were 6 times higher and deaths 12 times higher among those with underlying health conditions.[1] We understand the benefits of lifestyle modifications in preventing disease and reducing strain on the healthcare system. Improved health habits could even help ease the pressures that physicians face today regarding time constraints and limited resources. Furthermore, a healthy society is a productive society; companies are beginning to embrace the idea of encouraging better health in their workforce to both save money on company health plans and create more engaged employees.

Preventative efforts have been moderately successful in some realms. According to the CDC, the number of flu shots went up from 146.4 million during the 2015–2016 season to nearly 170 million during 2018–2019 season,[2] and the number of smokers in the United States declined 28.4 percent from 1965 to 2017.[3] However, despite the large amount of evidence supporting the benefits of lifestyle changes and the adoption of lifestyle medicine procedures and practices into virtually every evidence-based clinical guideline addressing chronic diseases (see Box 9.1), little progress has been made overall in improving the habits and practices of the American people.

Box 9.1   Clinical Guidelines from National Organizations That Incorporate Lifestyle Medicine Principles and Practices

- 2020 International Society of Hypertension Global Hypertension Practice Guidelines: U. Thomas, B. Claudio, C. Fadi, N.A. Khan, N.R. Poulter, D. Prabhakaran, A. Ramirez, M. Schlaich, G.S. Stergiou, M. Tomaszewski, R.D. Wainford, B. Williams, and A.E. Schutte, "2020 International Society of Hypertension Global Hypertension Practice Guidelines," *Hypertension* 75, no. 6 (June 1, 2020): 1334–1357. https://doi.org/10.1161/HYPERTENSIONAHA.120.15026
- Scientific Report of the 2020 Dietary Guidelines Advisory Committee: Dietary Guidelines Advisory Committee, *Scientific Report of the 2020 Dietary Guidelines Advisory Committee: Advisory Report to the Secretary of Agriculture and the Secretary of Health and Human Services* (Washington, DC: U.S. Department of Agriculture, Agricultural Research Service, 2020).
- American Academy of Pediatrics Guidelines on Primary Prevention of Obesity: S.R. Daniels, S.G. Hassink, and Committee On Nutrition, "The Role of the Pediatrician in Primary Prevention of Obesity," *Pediatrics*, 136, no. 1 (2015): e275–e292, https://doi.org/10.1542/peds.2015-1558.
- The American Heart Association 2030 Impact Goal: S.Y. Angell, M.V. McConnell, C. A.M. Anderson, D.S. Boyle, S. Capewell, M. Ezzati, S. de Ferranti, D.J. Gaskin, R.Z. Goetzel, M.D. Huffman, M. Jones, Y.M. Khan, S. Kim, S.K. Kumanyika, A.T. McCray, R.K. Merritt, B. Milstein, D. Mozaffarian, T. Norris, G.A. Roth, R.L. Sacco, J.F. Saucedo, C.M. Shay, D. Siedzik, S. Saha, and J.J. Warner, "The American Heart Association 2030 Impact Goal: A Presidential Advisory From the American Heart Association," *Circulation* 141, no. 9 (2020): e120–e138, https://doi.org/10.1161/CIR.0000000000000758.
- "Physical Activity Guidelines for Americans," 2nd ed. U.S. Department of Health and Human Services, https://health.gov/sites/default/files/2019-10/PAG_ExecutiveSummary.pdf.
- American Institute for Cancer Research Third Expert Report: World Cancer Research Fund/American Institute for Cancer Research, *Diet, Nutrition, Physical Activity and Cancer: A Global Perspective,* Continuous Update Project Expert Report, 2018, https://www.wcrf.org/dietandcancer.

- Defining Optimal Brain Health in Adults: A Presidential Advisory from the American Heart Association/American Stroke Association: P.B. Gorelick, K.L. Furie, C. Iadecola, E.E. Smith, S.P. Waddy, D.M. Lloyd-Jones, H.-J. Bae, M.A. Bauman, M. Dichgans, P.W. Duncan, M. Girgus, V.J. Howard, R.M. Lazar, S. Seshadri, F.D. Testai, S. van Gaal, K. Yaffe, H. Wasiak, and C. Zerna, "Defining Optimal Brain Health in Adults: A Presidential Advisory From the American Heart Association/American Stroke Association," *Stroke* 48, no. 10 (2017): e284–e303, https://doi.org/10.1161/STR.0000000000000148.

According to the CDC, 6 in 10 of adult Americans suffer from at least one chronic condition, defined broadly as conditions that last one year or more and require ongoing medical attention or limit activities of daily living or both, while 4 in 10 adult Americans suffer from at least two chronic conditions.[4] Furthermore, the number is projected to continue to grow as the population ages. Therefore, it is not surprising that 46 percent of all adult Americans and 90 percent of 65-year-old Americans and older take prescription medications.[4] In addition to the health costs to individuals and to society, the economics of chronic disease are unsustainable, and the solvency of our nation is at stake. Currently, 18 percent of the U.S. gross domestic product is spent on healthcare, and the CDC states that 90 percent of the nation's $3.5 trillion in annual health expenditures are spent on treating chronic diseases and mental health conditions.[5] By 2030, the World Economic Forum expects that the global burden of chronic diseases will grow to $47 trillion.[6] Box 9.2 lists data on the prevalence and economic impact of chronic diseases in the United States.

There is now a wide body of evidence that positive lifestyle factors can lower the incidence of chronic disease and promote general health. According to the World Health Organization (WHO), 80 percent of heart disease, stroke, and type 2 diabetes and 40 percent of cancer could be prevented primarily through improvements to lifestyle.[12] The Nurses' Health Study found that 80 percent of all heart disease and over 91 percent of all diabetes in women could be eliminated by adopting a cluster of positive lifestyle practices, including maintaining a healthy body weight, engaging in regular physical activity, not smoking cigarettes, and following a few simple nutritional guidelines.[13] The U.S. Health Professionals Study found similar reductions in chronic disease risk in men from the same lifestyle factors and even

---

Box 9.2 Statistics of Chronic Disease Prevalence and Economic Impact in the United States

---

- Chronic diseases are the leading cause of death and disability.[7]
- Six in 10 adult Americans suffer from at least one chronic condition.
- Four in 10 adult Americans suffer from at least two chronic conditions.
- Over two-thirds of the adult population is overweight or obese.[8]
- Approximately 45 percent of the adult population has high blood pressure.[9]
- Over 80 percent of the adult population does not get enough physical activity to result in health benefits.[10]
- The United States spends 18 percent of its gross domestic product on healthcare, of which 90 percent is spent on treating chronic diseases and mental health conditions.
- Costs of diet-related diseases, including diabetes, cardiovascular diseases, obesity-related cancers, and other obesity-related conditions are estimated to be $1.72 trillion per year.[11]
- All projections point to a continued rise in rates of chronic disease.

---

found that the risk of developing coronary artery disease would drop by half if just one of these positive lifestyle factors were adopted.[14]

Physicians have long espoused the practice of evidence-based medicine. Yet despite the vast body of evidence supporting the efficacy of lifestyle-based interventions on promoting positive health outcomes, the medical community has been slow to react. U.S. medical schools provide on average only 19.6 hours of required teaching about nutrition, with only 27 percent of schools providing the bare minimum of 25 hours set out by the National Academy of Sciences in 1985.[15] A systematic review published in 2019 found that "nutrition is insufficiently incorporated into medical education, regardless of country, setting, or year of medical education."[16p385] Furthermore, the current fee-for-service healthcare model in the United States does not incentivize cost savings and healthy outcomes but rather puts pressure on physicians to see as many patients as possible. Instead of encouraging physicians to focus on preventing diseases, physicians are forced to make quick diagnoses and send patients home with prescriptions to treat diseases when they arise.

The fee-for-service model is potentially contributing to the physician burnout epidemic (see Chapter 10 of this volume). Most physicians enter medicine with a high level of altruism and internal motivation and are likely to be significantly far along the stages of moral and psychosocial development (see Chapter 1 of this volume). Intrinsic motivators that allow physicians to find meaning in their work are likely to be valuable sources of joy and satification and, as such, for preventing burnout.[17] However, healthcare policymakers misguidedly continue to place extrinsic motivators on physicians that actually work to strip away instrinsic motivation. For example, our work is translated into relative value units for compensation purposes. While physicians want to spend time with patients and deliver patient-centered care, the system tends to prioritize metrics and money. A model of medicine that aims to treat the whole patient, focusing on prevention, may be part of the solution for physicians to rediscover meaning in their work.

To address the need for a therapeutic modality that empowers patients to protect their health, prevent diseases, and even treat and reverse diseases through lifestyle choices, the field of *lifestyle medicine* was created. The pioneers in the field of lifestyle medicine include T. Colin Campbell, Garry Egger, Caldwell Esselstyn Jr., Michael Greger, David L. Katz, John McDougall, Dean Ornish, Nathan Pritkin, and James Rippe. In the book, *Lifestyle Medicine*, James Rippe described lifestyle medicine as "the discipline of studying how daily habits and practices impact both on the prevention and treatment of disease, often in conjunction with pharmaceutical or surgical therapy, to provide an important adjunct to overall health." [18,pxiv] Although many medical organizations incorporate the values of lifestyle medicine, it is now evident that a centralized effort to improve health through lifestyle practices is needed. To meet this need, representatives from a variety of organizations including the American Academy of Pediatrics, the American College of Sports Medicine, the Academy of Nutrition and Dietetics, the American Academy of Family Practice, and the American College of Preventive Medicine established the first summary of competencies physicians should possess to practice lifestyle medicine.[19] Furthermore, the American College of Lifestyle Medicine (ACLM) was formed as a professional organization for physicians and other health professionals dedicated to the practice of lifestyle medicine as a foundation of a transformed and sustainable healthcare system. Practice of lifestyle medicine is different from preventive medicine, which is a field more focused on public health. Lifestyle medicine involves the use of evidence-based therapeutic approaches, such as eating a pre-dominantly whole food, plant-based diet, getting regular physical activity, adequate sleep, managing stress, avoiding use of risky substances, and pursuing other nondrug modalities to treat, reverse, and prevent chronic disease.[20] The ACLM is now one of the fastest-growing professional medical organizations.

It is crucial for medical professionals to understand the importance of lifestyle choices not only for the health of their patients but also for their personal well-being. In October 2017, the World Medical Association—an international confederation of more than 10 million physicians from 114 nations—unanimously voted to revise the Geneva Declaration, a modern successor to the Hippocratic Oath, to include the clause, "I will attend to my own health, well-being, and abilities in order to provide care of the highest standard."[21p1971] As we described in Chapter 3 of this volume, self-care ought to be a priority for physicians. Self-care includes lifestyle practices such as healthy eating and getting enough physical activity and sleep. Just as we must first put on our own oxygen mask before we can help others, we ought to focus on our health and happiness in order to help patients more effectively. Furthermore, evidence shows that physicians who are more confident in their own lifestyle practices are more likely to discuss lifestyle interventions with their patients.[22]

In the reminder of this chapter, we will discuss how one of the most prominent chronic diseases, obesity, is underscoring the need for lifestyle medicine. We then provide a brief overview of six key aspects of lifestyle habits and practices, described as the Six Pillars of Lifestyle Medicine by the ACLM, and discuss how these pillars can help reverse the trends of chronic disease in the United States and improve the well-being of medical professionals and their patients.

Lifestyle medicine as a response to the obesity crisis

Obesity is becoming a growing concern in the United States, and systematic efforts have yet to make a dramatic impact in stemming the tide. The causes are complex: genetics, the newfound availability of calorically dense foods, work-related stress, and lobbying efforts by "Big Food" have all contributed to the rising trend of obesity. In 2019, the CDC reported that from 1999–2000 through 2017–2018, the prevalence of obesity in adults aged 20 and over increased from 30.5 percent to 42.4 percent, and the prevalence of severe obesity increased from 4.7 percent to 9.2 percent.[23] Obesity and obesity-related diseases—such as heart disease, stroke, type 2 diabetes, and certain types of cancer—represent one of the leading causes of preventable death in the United States. Furthermore, obesity and its related diseases have been estimated to account for $190 billion per year of healthcare spending, approximately 21 percent of all United States healthcare expenditures.[24]

The complexity of providing care for obesity is of particular concern to physicians. One potential barrier is limitations placed by insurance providers on certain interventions for obese patients, including bariatric surgery. As an example, one insurance carrier requires that a patient is diagnosed with class 3 obesity (body mass index of over 40) for at least two years before covering bariatric surgery.[25] They further stipulate that patients with a body mass index of at least 35 can still qualify if they have the following conditions for which bariatric surgery could be an effective method of treatment: type 2 diabetes mellitus, coronary heart disease, clinically obstructive sleep apnea, and medically refractory hypertension. However, once a patient meets these restrictions, they must also prove that they have attempted weight loss in the past without successful long-term weight reduction and participate in either a physician-supervised nutrition and exercise program or a multidisciplinary surgical preparatory regimen.[26]

Obese patients face other barriers to care. Standard magnetic resonance imaging and computed tomography machines, which are tremendously useful in diagnosing many conditions, are not designed to accommodate patients above a defined weight limit. The popular press oftentimes reports examples of incidents, such as the story of a woman who was forced to weigh herself at a junkyard because her doctor's scale could not accommodate her and an incident where an obese patient was sent to the local zoo to complete an imaging procedure.[27] Although horrendous accounts such as these exist, many hospitals have updated their hardware to treat morbidly obese patients. Manufacturers have begun to produce open diagnostic imaging machines that are able to generate superior quality images of patients who before could not fit into an magnetic resonance imaging or computed tomography machine.

Unfortunately, these new technologies are purely reactionary and a response to the failure of preventative methods to stem the tide of obesity. Can we, as physicians, be content to treat only the symptoms and not the cause of this epidemic? Physicians have a duty not only to assuage the pain and suffering of those who are overweight but also to try to prevent medical diseases before they begin. Remember that we live in a society with limited resources, and it is a tenet of professionalism to use scarce capital equitably. One way to do this is to use fewer resources to prevent problems, which will be more costly down the road. This is one of the goals of lifestyle medicine.

The global context of the obesity crisis

Although the obesity problem is often framed as an American crisis or at least one that only affects a small subset of the world's wealthiest countries, this is no longer the case. According to the WHO, worldwide obesity tripled between 1975 and 2016.[28] Most of the world's population now lives in countries where being overweight and obesity is responsible for more deaths than illness associated with being underweight. And even in low- and middle-income countries— in which communicable diseases are still a major issue and undernutrition is still lurking—obesity also challenges the health of citizens. The WHO notes that children in these countries are more likely not to have their nutritional needs met even as they gain weight from high-sugar, high-fat, high-salt, and micronutrient-poor foods and that undernutrition and obesity can exist even within the same household.

It is no coincidence that global obesity trends have begun to parallel obesity trends in America. As Western companies and ideals spread around the world, so too do our unhealthy habits. As low- and middle-income countries continue to modernize, their citizens begin facing the same obstacles to a healthy diet and lifestyle that people in the United States have in recent decades. People move away from the social support of rural areas to the stress of finding a job in the city and making ends meet, and this stress leads to weight gain. This stress, combined with the city culture and long hours on the job, leads to sleep deprivation, which contributes to more weight gain. The American, meat-heavy diet has become a model for many other countries, whose people traditionally ate grains or other foods. Other parts of the American diet, including junk food and sugary drinks, are exported and advertised around the world. It seems that nowhere is safe from the lifestyle changes that have caused poor health in the United States.

There is a wealth of research of the root causes for the obesity epidemic. However, a systemic effort to educate physicians on the causes of chronic diseases such as obesity, as well as training on how exactly to engage in preventative medicine effectively with patients, is necessary to leverage this information and fulfill our responsibilities.

How can we address the obesity crisis?

Like the aggressive anti-tobacco advertising campaigns that have been effective for reducing the prevalence of smoking,[29] similar anti-obesity campaigns have been launched.[30] However, there has been far more criticism for these intense, no-holds barred, anti-obesity campaigns, especially those involving children. Critics claim that the advertisements merely ostracize and belittle overweight and obese people without offering any solution to the problem.[31] Because weight gain and weight loss are complex issues that involve diet, lifestyle, genetics, and physiological processes, these commercials may not be as effective as crusades against addiction. Merely informing people about the issue is not enough to affect change. We must find some way of getting the message across that will motivate people to alter their lifestyles for good.

The criticisms against anti-obesity campaigns may hold some merit. A longitudinal study reports a correlation between participants' perceived levels of physical activity and mortality.[32] Interestingly, study participants who reported above average to average levels of physical activity but actually had below average activity levels *did not* have an increased risk of mortality, while those who reported below average activity but had average or above average levels *did*. Thus, positive or negative expectations regarding one's health outcomes could potentially produce a physiological response by contributing placebo or nocebo effects. The implication for healthcare professionals and anti-obesity campaigns is that a more positive and motivational approach to obesity interventions could prove more effective than anti-obesity programming. Education about the benefits of pre-existing healthy lifestyle choices such as exercise and healthy eating can reinforce and potentially increase these behaviors, allowing propagation and reaping of full benefits. Of course, there is a fine line between constructive feedback that leads to the improvement of health outcomes and an overly complacent approach that leads to stagnation. Physicians must keep these considerations of perception and affect in mind to devise a tactful yet effective approach to treating obese patients, as well as other patients suffering from chronic symptoms.

Research shows that different words used by physicians to address weight concerns have a differential effect on patients' perception of the words as motivational, blaming, or stigmatizing. One survey of American adult patients found that words like *fat, obese,* and *morbidly obese* were perceived as undesirable because the patients felt like they were being blamed and stigmatized.[33] In contrast, the words *unhealthy weight* and *overweight* provided the most motivation for patients to lose weight. This illustrates the importance of tact in addressing changes to diet and lifestyle. Furthermore, 19 percent of the patients responded that they would avoid future medical appointments if they felt stigmatized by the physician, 21 percent would find a different physician, and 13 to 18 percent would feel less motivated and eat more food.

Potential interventions for chronic diseases: the Six Pillars of Lifestyle Medicine

Lifestyle medicine focuses on six evidence-based lifestyle modifications to improve health and combat chronic disease:

1. Healthful eating
2. Increasing physical activity
3. Improving sleep
4. Managing stress
5. Avoiding risky substances
6. Forming and maintaining relationships

These are called the Six Pillars of Lifestyle Medicine (see Figure 9.1). Of the six pillars, we have discussed in this volume the importance of social connections in Chapter 3 and will discuss in greater detail stress management strategies in Chapter 10 and substance use disorders in Chapter 12.

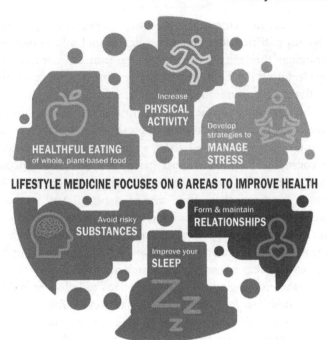

Figure 9.1 The six pillars of lifestyle medicine.
From https://lifestylemedicine.org/What-is-Lifestyle-Medicine. Used by permission.

Nutrition

You can't compete with what you eat.

Nutrition is often one of the most controversial and difficult subjects for healthcare providers to address. Food plays a prominent role in our lives, affecting us in the physical, social, emotional, and even spiritual levels. Nevertheless, regardless of individual factors, there is consistent and compelling evidence to support that healthy eating patterns can prevent, halt, and reverse diseases. However, there is a lack of education and lack of consistent guidelines on proper nutrition. What should we eat, and how much of it? There are many conflicting sources of information on this topic.

Whereas physicians should be leaders in communicating evidence-based information about nutrition to their patients, they aren't receiving the appropriate education. One study found that 22 percent of physicians did not receive any nutrition education in medical school, and 35 percent stated that the extent of their nutrition education was from a single lecture or part of a single lecture.[34] Furthermore, only 21 percent of patients felt that they received effective communication about nutrition from their physicians.

What, then, are the basic facts about nutrition that physicians ought to know? The concept of nutritional status represents the "bodily state resulting from the intake, absorption, utilization, and metabolism of the diet the individual consumes."[35p78] "Nutritional status" is a term that encompasses many components, often summarized with an acronym, the ABCDEFs: anthropometry, biochemical markers, clinical status, dietary intake, energy expenditure, and functional status.[36] Genetics are another component that affect nutritional status. As personalized nutrition develops, we may be able to address more of these determinants. However, as of now, dietary intake is the main factor that can be easily assessed and modified.

What are the proper guidelines for physicians to follow regarding diet? The *Dietary Guidelines for Americans* is updated every five years to reflect the current body of literature and provides evidence-based practices for Americans to improve their health. The most recent edition, from 2015 to 2020, provides five overarching guidelines:[37]

1. Follow a healthy eating pattern across the lifespan.
2. Focus on variety, nutrient density, and amount.
3. Limit calories from added sugars and saturated fats and reduce sodium intake.
4. Shift to healthier food and beverage choices.
5. Support healthy eating patterns for all.

According to the *Dietary Guidelines*, about three-fourths of the American population has a diet that is low in vegetables and fruits. More than half of the population meets or exceeds total grain and total protein recommendations but does not meet the recommendations for subgroups within each. Most of the population exceeds the recommendations of added sugars, saturated fats, and sodium. Certain shifts within and across food groups would benefit most individuals. Some of these shifts are minor and can be accomplished through making simple substitutions, while others require greater effort to accomplish. Nevertheless, we have a responsibility to communicate the value of these nutritional modifications.

Changing the nutritional habits of the general populace is not solely the responsibility of physicians. Collective action is needed across all segments of society to improve nutrition. Actions must involve identifying successful approaches for change, improving knowledge of what constitutes healthy eating, enhancing access to healthy and affordable food choices, and promoting change in social and cultural norms to embrace healthy lifestyle practices.

Increase physical activity

Those who regularly practice physical activity "carry a lower risk of premature mortality and of contracting several of the most prevalent chronic diseases."[38p177] Physical activity has a myriad of documented health benefits. It protects against excessive weight gain, and has been shown to be associated with improved quality of life through improvements in sleep quality and feelings of general well-being. Physical activity has also been shown to be associated with lower incidence rates of cancer, as well as increased cognitive function and reduced feelings of anxiety and depression.

The Physical Activity Guidelines for Americans, updated by the U.S. Department of Health and Human Services in 2018, recommends that adults participate in 150 to 300 minutes of moderate-intensity physical activity or 75 to 150 minutes of vigorous-intensity physical activity per week.[39] These guidelines also state that muscle-strengthening exercise should also be practiced two to three days per week. Everyone should be physically active, and if these guidelines cannot be satisfied due to medical conditions or frailty, they should be attained to the best of one's ability.

Approximately 80 percent of U.S. adults and adolescents are insufficiently active, making it a prominent risk factor for chronic diseases. Alarmingly, it has been estimated that less than 40 percent of physicians regularly counsel their patients on the value of exercise and physical activity.[40] As medical professionals, we are able to play a vital role in convincing patients to make lifestyle changes by providing specific and individualized exercise recommendations.

Sleep

Sleep quality is not something that is routinely assessed in a physical exam, but it has huge implications on health and well-being. Many studies have shown that decreased sleep duration and poor sleep quality are linked to chronic diseases.[41] Physicians should take steps to communicate with patients the benefits of a good night's sleep. Sleep loss has a host of effects on the body, including alterations in neuroendocrine function and glucose metabolism. Experiments have shown that sleep-deprived subjects exhibit lower levels of the satiety hormone leptin and higher levels of the appetite-stimulating hormone ghrelin,[42] which can lead to overeating through increased hunger response. Yet another harmful effect of sleep loss is decreased sensitivity to insulin, making it a risk factor for the development of type 2 diabetes.[43] Sleep deprivation has also been shown to be associated with increased blood pressure,[44] decreased immune function,[45] and increased risk for depression and anxiety.[46]

While inadequate sleep has become more prevalent due to the demands of modern society, it is not usually addressed as an important aspect of lifestyle that can and should be modified. Working long hours and sleeping little is often seen as a requirement or a laudable activity. However, according to the National Institutes of Health, people who suffer from sleep deficiency are even "less productive at work and school, take longer to finish tasks, have a slower reaction time, and make more mistakes."[47] We can work to change societal perceptions about the importance of sleep. As physicians, we have a responsibility to counsel patients on the proper guidelines and habits.

Stress

According to the constitution of the WHO, "health is a state of complete physical, mental, and social well-being and not merely the absence of disease or infirmity."[48p984] Managing stress effectively to maintain well-being is therefore an essential part of a healthy lifestyle. The first step of stress management is to identify stressors in a process called cognitive appraisal. Then, coping strategies may be used to form positive responses to stress, allowing us to maintain our emotional well-being even during challenging situations. Coping strategies can either be adaptive or avoidant, referring to whether or not the strategy seeks to reframe stressors, or avoid them altogether. Common coping strategies include mindfulness, deep breathing, meditation, music therapy, and exercise. Stress and coping strategies are discussed in more detail in Chapter 10 of this volume.

Substance use

Substance use represents one of the most significant factors leading to premature death in the United States. Substance use disorders also contribute to significant medical and psychiatric complications that contribute to decreased quality of life and economic burden. Tobacco continues to significantly contribute to morbidity and mortality, even as rates of tobacco use have declined significantly over the past few decades. Alcohol is another commonly used substance that contributes to chronic diseases. According to the 2018 National Survey on Drug Use and Health, 86.3 percent of people ages 18 or older reported that they drank alcohol at some point in their lifetime, with 14.4 million adults ages 18 and older suffering from alcohol use disorder.[49] The use of illicit drugs, such as heroin and cocaine, and abuse of prescriptions drugs, such as oxycodone and benzodiazepines, have also led to unprecedented statistics of morbidity and mortality.[50]

Despite the prevalence of substance use disorders in the United States, treatment has not been adequate. Substance use disorders have often been viewed as the result of moral failings or criminal behavior, and healthcare providers have not received adequate education on how to assist patients suffering from substance use disorders. Treatment of substance use disorders requires ongoing treatment and management and requires that the patient be engaged with their own treatment. Substance use disorder are discussed in more detail in Chapter 12 of this volume.

Relationships

The landmark Harvard Study of Adult Development found that the quality of our relationships has a profound effect on our health.[51] Healthy relationships can help protect us from stress, delay mental and physical decline, and increase feelings of contentment and satisfaction with life. On the other hand, social isolation is associated with adverse health consequences, including depression, poor sleep quality, impaired executive function, accelerated cognitive decline, poor cardiovascular function and impaired immunity, as well as risk of premature death.[52] In the PERMA model of well-being (see Chapter 3 of this volume), healthy relationships are one of the main components of well-being. Therefore, encouraging healthy relationships for our patients is a vital aspect of lifestyle medicine.

Physicians attending to their own wellness

One of the tenets of medical professionalism is to attend to our own well-being and health through self-care. Due to the demands of the profession, maintaining a healthy lifestyle is particularly challenging for physicians and other health professionals. Impediments against developing and maintaining healthy habits include long work hours and little time to exercise, prepare food, and sleep. Furthermore, the "culture of silence" prevalent among health professionals can make it difficult for physicians to seek help or be open about their feelings and struggles regarding lifestyle choices.[53] The high-pressure environment that medical students, residents, and physicians find themselves in is often not conducive to seeking professional help.[54] Personality traits common among physicians such as perfectionism and mental rigidity, coupled with environmental stressors, are likely to intensify unhealthy lifestyle practices.[55]

Relatively scarce data exist regarding the prevalence of unhealthy lifestyle practices and chronic disorders within the physician population, but evidence suggests that physicians fare no better than the general population. In a survey of physicians in California, 35 percent of participants reported "no" or "occasional" exercise.[56] Furthermore, 34 percent reported six or fewer hours of sleep per night, and 21 percent reported working more than 60 hours per week. Prevalence of physician burnout, as well as depression and other chronic disorders and diseases, are likely tied to lifestyle practices.

Could unhealthy lifestyle choices among medical professionals largely be due to lack of education and inadequate resources? Educational institutions often struggle to address the growing body of evidence that espouses the importance of nutrition, exercise, and sleep, among other facets of lifestyle, on well-being. Furthermore, long, erratic hours, and the inaccessibility of fresh, whole food options at work may be contributing significantly to the prevalence of obesity and type 2 diabetes, as well as burnout and other chronic conditions among physicians. The issues are largely systemic, but we can at least work to modify the factors that we are able to control and facilitate development of a healthy lifestyle environment.

Chapter Quick Summary

- Lifestyle habits and actions have a tremendous impact on our health and quality of life, particularly in preventing and abating chronic disease.
- Limited education is currently given in medical training on the importance of lifestyle on preventing disease.
- Chronic disease is an epidemic in the United States that is only projected to get worse as the population ages, with the solvency of our nation at stake.
- Two of the most prominent chronic diseases in the United States, obesity and diabetes, underscore the need for lifestyle medicine.
- The American College of Lifestyle Medicine espouses six evidence-based lifestyle interventions for improving health, called the Six Pillars: healthful eating, increasing physical activity, improving sleep, managing stress, avoiding risky substances, and forming and maintaining relationships.

Resources

American College of Lifestyle Medicine. "Lifestyle Medicine: Scientific Evidence." https://www.lifestylemedicine.org/ACLM/Lifestyle_Medicine/Scientific_Evidence/ACLM/About/What_is_Lifestyle_Medicine_/Scientific_Evidence.aspx?hkey=ed4b4130-6ce9-41bb-8703-211bc98eed7f

American Journal of Lifestyle Medicine. [Home page]. https://journals.sagepub.com/home/ajl

Campbell, T.C., and T.H. Campbell II. *The China Study: Revised and Expanded Edition: The Most Comprehensive Study of Nutrition Ever Conducted and the*

Startling Implications for Diet, Weight Loss, and Long-Term Health. Rev. ed. Dallas, TX: BenBella Books, 2016.

Esselstyn, C.B., Jr. *Prevent and Reverse Heart Disease: The Revolutionary, Scientifically Proven, Nutrition-Based Cure*. 1st ed. New York: Avery, 2008.

Greger, M., and G. Stone. *How Not to Die: Discover the Foods Scientifically Proven to Prevent and Reverse Disease*. 1st ed. New York: Flatiron Books, 2015.

Ornish, D., and A. Ornish. *Undo It! How Simple Lifestyle Changes Can Reverse Most Chronic Diseases*. Ill. ed. New York: Ballantine Books, 2019.

References

1. Stokes, E.K., L.D. Zambrano, K.N. Anderson, E.P. Marder, K.M. Raz, S. El Burai Felix, Y. Tie, and K.E. Fullerton. "Coronavirus Disease 2019 Case Surveillance— United States, January 22–May 30, 2020." *Morb Mortal Wkly Rep* 69, no. 24 (2020): 759–765. http://dx.doi.org/10.15585/mmwr.mm6924e2

2. Centers for Disease Control and Prevention. "2015–16 Seasonal Influenza Vaccine Total Doses Distributed." March 3, 2016. https://www.cdc.gov/flu/prevent/vaccinesupply-2015.html

3. Centers for Disease Control and Prevention. "Smoking Is Down, but Almost 38 Million American Adults Still Smoke." November 11, 2018. https://www.cnbc.com/2018/11/08/cdc-says-smoking-rates-fall-to-record-low-in-us.html

4. Centers for Disease Control and Prevention. "About Chronic Diseases." 2020. https://www.cdc.gov/chronicdisease/about/index.htm

5. Centers for Disease Control and Prevention. "Health and Economic Costs of Chronic Diseases." 2020. https://www.cdc.gov/chronicdisease/about/costs/index.htm

6. Bloom, D.E., E. Cafiero, E. Jané-Llopis, S. Abrahams-Gessel, L.R. Bloom, S. Fathima, A.B. Feigl, T. Gaziano, A. Hamandi, M. Mowafi, D. O'Farrell, E. Ozaltin, A. Pandya, K. Prettner, L. Rosenberg, B. Seligman, A.Z. Stein, C. Weinstein, and J. Weiss. "The Global Economic Burden of Noncommunicable Diseases." PGDA Working Papers 8712, Program on the Global Demography of Aging. 2012. http://www.hsph.harvard.edu/pgda/WorkingPapers/2012/PGDA_WP_87.pdf

7. Raghupathi, W., and V. Raghupathi. "An Empirical Study of Chronic Diseases in the United States: A Visual Analytics Approach to Public Health." *Int J Environ Res Public Health* 15, no. 3 (2018): 431. https://doi.org/10.3390/ijerph15030431

8. National Center for Health Statistics. "Obesity and Overweight." 2020. https://www.cdc.gov/nchs/fastats/obesity-overweight.htm

9. Centers for Disease Control and Prevention. "Facts about Hypertension." 2020. https://www.cdc.gov/bloodpressure/facts.htm

10. Piercy, K.L., R.P. Troiano, R.M. Ballard, S.A. Carlson, J.E. Fulton, D.A. Galuska, S.M. George, and R.D. Olson. "The Physical Activity Guidelines for Americans." *JAMA* 320, no. 19 (2018): 2020–228. https://doi.org/10.1001/jama.2018.14854

11. Waters, H., and G. Marlon. "America's Obesity Crisis: The Health and Economic Costs of Excess Weight." *Milken Institute*. 2018. https://milkeninstitute.org/reports/americas-obesity-crisis-health-and-economic-costs-excess-weight

12. World Health Organization. "Preventing Chronic Diseases: A Vital Investment." 2015. https://www.who.int/chp/chronic_disease_report/en/

13. Liu, S., M.J. Stampfer, F.B. Hu, E. Giovannucci, E. Rimm, J.E. Manson, C.H. Hennekens, and W.C. Willett. "Whole-Grain Consumption and Risk of Coronary Heart Disease: Results from the Nurses' Health Study." *Am J Clin Nutr* 70, no. 3 (1999): 412–419. https://doi.org/10.1093/ajcn/70.3.412

14. Chiuve, S.E., M.L. McCullough, F.M. Sacks, and E.B. Rimm. "Healthy Lifestyle Factors in the Primary Prevention of Coronary Heart Disease among Men: Benefits among Users and Nonusers of Lipid-lowering and Antihypertensive Medications." *Circulation* 114, no. 2 (2006): 160–167. https://doi.org/10.1161/CIRCULATIONAHA.106.621417

15. Adams, K.M., M. Kohlmeier, and S.H. Zeisel. "Nutrition Education in U.S. Medical Schools: Latest Update of a National Survey." *Acad Med* 85, no. 9 (2010): 1537–1542. https://doi.org/10.1097/ACM.0b013e3181eab71b

16. Crowley, J., L. Ball, and G.J. Hiddink. "Nutrition in Medical Education: A Systematic Review." *Lancet Planet Health* 3, no. 9 (2019): e379–e389. https://doi.org/10.1016/S2542-5196(19)30171-8

17. Hartzband, P., and J. Groopman. "Physician Burnout, Interrupted." *New Eng J Med* 382, no. 26 (2020): 2485–2487. https://doi.org/10.1056/NEJMp2003149

18. Rippe, J.M., ed. *Lifestyle Medicine*. 3rd ed. Boca Raton: CRC Press, 2019.

19. Lianov, L., and M. Johnson. "Physician Competencies for Prescribing Lifestyle Medicine." *JAMA* 304, no. 2 (2010): 202–203. https://doi.org/10.1001/jama.2010.903

20. American College of Lifestyle Medicine. "Mission/Vision." 2019. https://www.lifestylemedicine.org/ACLM/About/Mission_Vision/ACLM/About/Mission_Vision.aspx?hkey=0c26bcd1-f424-416a-9055-2e3af80777f6

21. Parsa-Parsi, R.W. "The Revised Declaration of Geneva: A Modern-Day Physician's Pledge." *JAMA* 318, no. 20 (2017): 1971–1972. https://doi.org/10.1001/jama.2017.16230

22. Howe, M., A. Leidel, S.M. Krishnan, A. Weber, M. Rubenfire, and E.A. Jackson. "Patient-Related Diet and Exercise Counseling: Do Providers' Own Lifestyle Habits Matter?" *Prev Cardiol* 13, no. 4 (2010): 180–185. https://doi.org/10.1111/j.1751-7141.2010.00079.x

23. Hales, C.M., M.D. Carroll, C.D. Fryar, and C.L. Ogden. "Prevalence of Obesity and Severe Obesity among Adults: United States, 2017–2018." *NCHS Data Brief* 360. February 2020. https://www.cdc.gov/nchs/data/databriefs/db360-h.pdf

24. Cawley, J., and C. Meyerhoefer. "The Medical Care Costs of Obesity: An Instrumental Variables Approach." *J Health Econ* 31, no. 1 (2012): 219–230. https://doi.org/10.1016/j.jhealeco.2011.10.003

25. Aetna. "Obesity Surgery." Aetna Medical Clinical Policy Bulletin 0157. May 18, 2020. http://www.aetna.com/cpb/medical/data/100_199/0157.html

26. Ontario Medical Advisory Secretariat. "Bariatric Surgery: An Evidence-Based Analysis." *Ontario Health Technology Assessment Series* 5, no. 1 (2005): 1–148.

27. Kolata, G. "Why Do Obese Patients Get Worse Care? Many Doctors Don't See Past the Fat." *New York Times*. September 26, 2016. https://www.nytimes.com/2016/09/26/health/obese-patients-health-care.html?mcubz=2

28. World Health Organization. "Obesity and Overweight Factsheet." April 1, 2020. https://www.who.int/news-room/fact-sheets/detail/obesity-and-overweight

29. Duke, J.C., K.C. Davis, R.L. Alexander, A.J. MacMonegle, J.L. Fraze, R.M. Rodes, and D.M. Beistle. "Impact of a U.S. Antismoking National Media Campaign on Beliefs, Cognitions and Quit Intentions." *Health Educ Res* 30, no. 3 (2015): 466–483. https://doi.org/10.1093/her/cyv017

30. Emery, S.L., G. Szczypka, L.M. Powell, and F.J. Chaloupka. "Public Health Obesity-Related TV Advertising: Lessons Learned from Tobacco." *Am J Preven Med* 33, no. 4, suppl. (2007): S257–S263. https://doi.org/10.1016/j.amepre.2007.07.003

31. Puhl, R., J.L. Peterson, and J. Luedicke. "Fighting Obesity or Obese Persons? Public Perceptions of Obesity-related Health Messages." *Int J Obes* 37, no. 6 (2013): 774–782. https://doi.org/10.1038/ijo.2012.156

32. Zahrt, O.H., and A.J. Crum. "Perceived Physical Activity and Mortality: Evidence from Three Nationally Representative US Samples." *Health Psychol* 36, no. 11 (2017): 1017.

33. Puhl, R., J.L. Peterson, and J. Luedicke. "Motivating or Stigmatizing? Public Perceptions of Weight-related Language Used by Health Providers." *Int J Obes* 37, no. 4 (2013): 612–619. https://doi.org/10.1038/ijo.2012.110

34. Aggarwal, M., S. Devries, A.M. Freeman, R. Ostfeld, H. Gaggin, P. Taub, A.K. Rzeszut, K. Allen, and R.C. Conti. "The Deficit of Nutrition Education of Physicians." *Am J Med* 131, no. 4 (2018): 339–345. https://doi.org/10.1016/j.amjmed.2017.11.036

35. Dwyer, J.T., and R.L. Bailey. "The Concept of Nutritional Status and it's Measurement." In *Lifestyle Medicine*. 3rd ed. Edited by J.M. Rippe, 77–100. Boca Raton, FL: CRC Press, 2019.

36. Madden, A., and R. Hoffman. "Assessment of nutritional status." In *Manual of Dietetic Practice*. Edited by J. Gandy. New York: Wiley, 2019.

37. U.S. Department of Health and Human Services, Office of Disease Prevention and Health Promotion. "2015–2020 Dietary Guidelines for Americans." 8th ed. December 2015. https://health.gov/our-work/food-nutrition/2015-2020-dietary-guidelines

38. Davis, P.G. "Exercise Prescription for Apparently Healthy Individuals and for Special Populations Lifestyle Medicine." In Lifestyle Medicine. 3rd ed. Edited by J.M. Rippe, 177–189. Boca Raton, FL: CRC Press, 2019.

39. Piercy, K.L., R.P. Troiano, R.M. Ballard, S.A. Carlson, J.E. Fulton, D.A. Galuska, S.M. George, and R.D. Olson. "The Physical Activity Guidelines." *JAMA* 320, no. 19 (2018): 2020–2028.

40. Rippe, J.M. "Lifestyle Medicine: The Health Promoting Power of Daily Habits and Practices." *Am J Lifestyle Med* 12, no. 6 (2018): 499–512. https://doi.org/10.1177/1559827618785554

41. Cooper, C.B., E.V. Neufeld, B.A. Dolezal, and J.L. Martin. "Sleep Deprivation and Obesity in Adults: A Brief Narrative Review." *BMJ Open Sport Exer Med* 4, no. 1 (2018): e000392.

42. Hanlon, E.C., E. Tasali, R. Leproult, K.L. Stuhr, E. Doncheck, H. De Wit, C.J. Hillard, and E. Van Cauter. "Sleep Restriction Enhances the Daily Rhythm of Circulating Levels of Endocannabinoid 2-arachidonoylglycerol." *Sleep* 39, no. 3 (2016): 653–664.

43. Mesarwi, O., J. Polak, J. Jun, and V.Y. Polotsky. "Sleep Disorders and the Development of Insulin Resistance and Obesity." *Endocrin Metab Clin* 42, no. 3 (2013): 617–634. https://doi.org/10.1016/j.ecl.2013.05.001

44. Calhoun, D.A., and S.M. Harding. "Sleep and Hypertension." *Chest* 138, no. 2 (2010): 434–443. https://doi.org/10.1378/chest.09-2954

45. Besedovsky, L., T. Lange, and J. Born. "Sleep and Immune Function." *Pflug Arch Eur J Phy* 463, no. 1 (2012): 121–137. https://doi.org/10.1007/s00424-011-1044-0

46. Hamilton, N.A., C.A. Nelson, N. Stevens, and H. Kitzman. "Sleep and Psychological Well-Being." *Soc Ind Res* 82, no. 1 (2007): 147–163. https://doi.org/10.1007/s11205-006-9030-1

47. National Heart, Lung, and Blood Institute. "Sleep Deprivation and Deficiency." https://www.nhlbi.nih.gov/health-topics/sleep-deprivation-and-deficiency

48. International Health Conference. "Constitution of the World Health Organization, 1946." *B World Health Org* 80, no. 12 (2002): 983–984. https://apps.who.int/iris/handle/10665/268688

49. Substance Abuse and Mental Health Services Administration. "2018 National Survey on Drug Use and Health: Methodological Summary and Definitions." Center for Behavioral Health Statistics and Quality, 2019. https://www.samhsa.gov/data/

50. Nelson, L.S., D.N. Juurlink, and J. Perrone. "Addressing the Opioid Epidemic." *JAMA* 314, no. 14 (2015): 1453–1454. https://doi.org/10.1001/jama.2015.12397

51. Ghent, A. "The Happiness Effect." *B World Health Org* 89, no. 4 (2011): 246–247. https://doi.org/10.2471/BLT.11.020411

52. Cacioppo, J.T., and L.C. Hawkley. "Social Isolation and Health, with an Emphasis on Underlying Mechanisms." *Perspect Biol Med* 46, no. 3 (2013): S39–S52. https://doi.org/10.1353/pbm.2003.0063

53. Ross, C. "When the Healers are Hurting: Understanding Eating Disorders." *Psychol Today.* April 29, 2013. https://www.psychologytoday.com/us/blog/real-healing/201304/when-the-healers-are-hurting-understanding-eating-disorders

54. Bates Freed, B. "Physician: Starve Thyself. Are Eating Disorders the Last Taboo in the Medical World?" *MD Edge.* November 26, 2012. https://www.mdedge.com/rheumatologynews/article/56629/health-policy/physician-starve-thyself-are-eating-disorders-last

55. Eley, D.S., J. Leung, B.A. Hong, K.M. Cloninger, and C.R. Cloninger. "Identifying the Dominant Personality Profiles in Medical Students: Implications for Their Well-Being and Resilience." *PLoS One* 11, no. 8 (2016). https://doi.org/10.1371/journal.pone.0160028

56. Bazargan, M., M. Makar, S. Bazargan-Hejazi, C. Ani, and K.E. Wolf. "Preventive, Lifestyle, and Personal Health Behaviors among Physicians." *Acad Psych* 33, no. 4 (2009): 289–295. https://doi.org/10.1176/appi.ap.33.4.289

10
Stress, Burnout, and Coping Strategies

As physicians, we seek to deliver high-quality, compassionate, patient-centered care. This requires that our clinical workforce is functioning at the highest level. However, growing evidence suggests that physician well-being is being eroded in the professional setting. Burnout—a work-related syndrome characterized by emotional exhaustion, depersonalization, and a low sense of accomplishment from work—is prevalent among physicians, trainees, and students. Evidence suggests that burnout affects over half of all physicians and between 45 and 60 percent of medical students and residents in the United States.[1] Alarmingly, these numbers continue to rise. Burnout not only leads to increased physician dissatisfaction, higher rates of turn-over, increased likelihood to use substances, and higher rates of depression and suicide but also to higher rates of medical error and negative patient outcomes. Physician burnout is a public health concern and a problem that needs to be addressed, for the well-being of physicians and their patients alike.

A growing body of evidence suggests that burnout is a systemic issue. Changes to the healthcare landscape in how care is delivered, documented, and reimbursed has led to decreased autonomy, increased clerical workload, and decreased trust in the system. For example, the widespread adoption of electronic health records—and the resulting interference with physician-patient interactions and increased clerical burden (see Chapters 4 and 5 of this volume)—has been a frequently cited factor for the increase in burnout. An imbalance of job demands and the resources available to deal with them, compounded with administrative pressures and reimbursement models that incentivize seeing as many patients as possible, may be other factors. Furthermore, the increased demand for healthcare—which will only continue to grow as the rates of chronic disease increase in the United States—may also contribute to burnout, particularly when compounded with the shortage of health professionals that currently exists in many areas.

Because physician burnout is a systemic issue, a concerted effort by all stakeholders to modify the systems of healthcare will be required to address the roots of the problem. A systems approach to address physician burnout that focuses on improving the structure, organization, and culture of healthcare has been suggested by the National Academy of Medicine's Action Collaborative on Clinician Well-Being and Resilience.[2] Initiatives by healthcare institutions and policymakers to address burnout are also beginning to appear. Among these are the American Medical Association's Practice Transformation Initiative and STEPS Forward Program and formation of wellness committees in medical schools and residency programs across the country.[3]

Nevertheless, we are not powerless as individuals. As medical professionals, we also have a mandate to take care of ourselves. There are steps we can take to abate and adapt to the stresses of the professional environment and protect ourselves from burnout. Adaptation is a normal response that follows a new-found stimulus, and all physicians adapt to the stressors of the healthcare environment in one way or another. Crucially, though, adaptation can either be positive or negative; when we engage in maladaptive responses to occupational stress, we may be putting ourselves at risk for burnout. By developing an understanding that stress is normal and not any fault of our own and by training for adaptive and healthy coping responses, we may be able to develop resilience against burnout at the individual level.

The stress response

A theory of stress and adaptation was first developed by Hans Selye, who conceived the general adaptation syndrome model.[4] Selye suggested that the human body strives for homeostasis; when confronted with external stressors, it undergoes an adaptive response to maintain balance. The first stage is *alarm*, which mobilizes the sympathetic nervous system when confronted with a stressor. The next stage is *resistance*, in which the body's sympathetic response allows for an increased capacity to respond to stress. This stage, however, is metabolically demanding and cannot last long before the third stage and final stage of *exhaustion* or *recovery* sets in. If the stressor is improperly dealt with, for example through maladaptive responses, exhaustion causes the body to be unable to maintain normal function. Over time, as exhaustion from stressors compound, psychological well-being may be damaged, eventually leading to burnout or other chronic mental illnesses.

Stress also can lead to physiological damage. Increased cortisol associated with the stress response has been shown to lead to blood sugar imbalances, high blood pressure, loss of muscle tissue and bone density, lower immunity, and inflammatory responses, in addition to structural changes to the brain.[5] Because the stress response is centered in the hypothalamic–pituitary–adrenal axis, the chronic effects of stress exhaustion may cause significant damage to this important system of neuroendocrine activity that regulates the immune system, metabolic balance, and other biological processes. Indeed, chronic stress has even been shown to predict decreased grey matter volume in the hippocampus.[6] However, when appropriate coping measures are used, the stressor is able to be overcome or eliminated in the process of recovery, returning the body to a state of homeostasis. The general adaptation syndrome model of stress is depicted in Figure 10.1.

It is increasingly evident that the neural processes underlying stress and stress resilience are complex and involve the interaction of neurobiological, genetic, epigenetic, and environmental components.[7] There are also different types of stress. Selye classified stress into two types: *eustress* and *distress*. Eustress refers to positive stress that helps motivate individuals and improves performance. An example of eustress in the clinic could be the

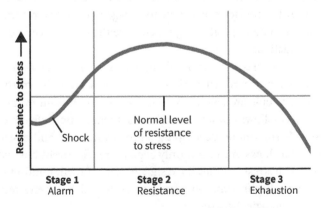

Figure 10.1 General adaptation syndrome model of stress.

challenges associated with coordinating a healthcare team to provide treatment for a complex disease. Eustress can lead to increased engagement or "flow," as described by positive psychologists.[8] Distress, on the other hand, tends to cause anxiety, decreases performance, and can lead to long-term exhaustion. Many of the systemic factors leading to widespread physician burnout could be classified as distress, such as decreased time to develop relationships with patients and decreased autonomy.

How can we learn to deal with distress? Richard Lazarus's transactional model of stress explains that when confronted with a stressor, we first undergo two forms of cognitive appraisal: *primary appraisal* identifies stimuli that are threatening to our well-being and *secondary appraisal* analyzes our ability to appropriately deal with the stressor with our available resources.[9] According to this model, evoking a particular coping response is not a direct response to the stressor but instead to the cognitive appraisal of the stressor. This means that by reframing our cognitive appraisal processes and developing healthy coping strategies that work for us individually, we can learn to adopt strategies to appropriately deal with stress.

A growth mindset and self-compassion can allow for positive cognitive restructuring. A *growth mindset*, defined by Carol Dweck, refers to a belief that one can acquire any given ability provided that they invest effort or study.[10] A growth mindset is in opposition to a *fixed mindset*, which views abilities as mostly innate and that failure is a representation of a lack of basic abilities. A growth mindset thrives on challenge and views failure as an opportunity for growth and is therefore able to more effectively deal with stress. By developing a growth mindset, one is able to engage in cognitive reappraisal to view stressors in a more positive light and have the confidence to deal with challenging situations.

Self-compassion has also been identified as an important element of this positive cognitive restructuring process. Research shows that self-compassionate people are less likely to catastrophize difficult events or experience anxiety following a stressor, allowing them to more effectively cope with stress.[11] Furthermore, developing a growth mindset and engaging in self-compassion allows one to not only cope more effectively, but even proactively deal with stress. Studies have shown that a growth mindset leads to decreased mental health symptoms and buffers the link between stressful life events and psychological distress.[12]

Coping with stress

Lazarus and Folkman provided the widely accepted definition of coping as thoughts and behaviors used by people to manage the internal and external demands of stressful situations.[9] Coping is a multidimensional process that is sensitive to the environment and the personal dimensions of the individual. Coping strategies have many forms, and classification of coping strategies into broad classifications has not been widely agreed upon. Lazarus and Folkman suggested a classification of *problem-based coping*, which aims to resolve the problem-causing distress, and *emotion-focused coping*, which aims to improve the negative emotions associated with a stressor.[9] An example of problem-based coping could be to develop a plan of action for avoiding a certain stressor, while an example of emotion-focused coping could be seeking out social support.

Evidence suggests that problem-based coping is linked with a greater sense of control, as well as a negative association with anxiety and depression.[13] These data agree with the concept of a growth mindset, as those who believe that stressors can be properly addressed are likely to engage in problem-based coping. On the other hand, emotion-based coping has been shown to be positively associated with anxiety and depression.[14] This is not to say, however, that problem-based coping is necessarily more effective than emotional-focused coping or that we should always seek to engage in problem-based coping strategies. Coping is highly individual and depends on the environment. For example, when the source of stress is entirely outside one's locus of control, emotion-based coping strategies such as mindfulness and meditation can be effective for dealing with the symptoms of stress.

Another common classification describes *approach* versus *avoidant coping*.[15] Approach, or active coping, is similar to problem-based coping in that it aims to address the underlying stressor. When applicable, these strategies tend to be effective long-term. Avoidant coping, on the other hand, includes behaviors that aim to reduce stress by distancing oneself from the problem.

After surveying and analyzing the literature, Skinner and colleagues identified over 400 different coping strategies, with five core categories of coping that are common among many classifications:

1. Positive cognitive restructuring.
2. Problem–solving.

3. Seeking support.
4. Distraction.
5. Escape/avoidance.[16-18]

Table 10.1 describes these five core categories of coping and examples of each.

Table 10.1 Five Core Categories of Coping

Categories of coping	Definition	Examples
Positive cognitive restructuring	Active attempts to change one's view of a stressful situation to see it in a more positive way	Positive thinking; focusing on the positive; optimism; minimization of distress or negative consequences
Problem solving	Strategies that seek to resolve the underlying stressor	Strategizing; planning; logical analysis; effort; persistence and determination
Seeking support	Asking for help from social contacts	Seeking support from parents, spouses, peers, professionals, and God with a variety of goals, including instrumental help, advice, comfort, and contact
Distraction	Active attempts to deal with a stressful situation by engaging in an alternative pleasurable activity	Engaging in hobbies; exercising; watching television; using social media; seeking friends; or reading
Escape/avoidance	Efforts to disengage or stay away from the stressful transaction	Cognitive avoidance; avoidant actions; denial and wishful thinking

Adapted from E.A. Skinner, K. Edge, J. Altman, and H. Sherwood, "Searching for the Structure of Coping: A Review and Critique of Category Systems for Classifying Ways of Coping," *Psychol Bull* 129, no. 2 (2003): 239–242, https://doi.org/10.1037/0033-2909.129.2.216. Used with permission.

Potential coping strategies for physicians

Many of the stresses that physicians face today in the workplace are no fault of our own and are largely out of our control. As a result, problem-solving or problem-based coping strategies may be difficult to implement. However, potential problem-solving initiatives could include delegating excessive responsibilities to other members of the healthcare team or creating to-do lists to stay on top of responsibilities. Learning to say "no" to voluntary responsibilities that you cannot handle is another valuable skill for maintaining well-being. However, there are several other strategies that we can take to mitigate stress and reduce risk for burnout.

Positive cognitive reconstruction using the ABC technique

Rather than feeling that our stress is our fault, we can work to develop an understanding that stress is normal and that we have the resilience to deal with it. Our medical culture tends to emphasize perfectionism and delayed gratification, traits that may actually be causing us undue anxiety and contributing to burnout. We can work to reframe our perspective to manage our expectations about stress, understand that being perfect is unattainable, and work toward personal happiness each day of our lives.

One method to accomplish this goal is to use the ABC technique from cognitive behavioral therapy.[19] The ABC technique, created by Albert Ellis, and later adopted by Martin Seligman, is a method for analyzing past events to which someone has had an emotional response. It requires review of past events and the recognition of a cause-and-effect relationship. The "A" stands for the *activating event*, and it can be anything that produces some sort of negative emotion. The "B" refers to our *beliefs*, which are influenced by the activating event. Finally, the "C" represents the *consequences* that we face because of how our beliefs color our response to the activating event. These consequences can be emotional or behavioral. The ABC technique focuses on the space between B and C, causing us to identify and reflect on our beliefs, recognize that that they may be irrational, and modify them to reshape the consequences. This is similar to the development of a growth mindset, allowing us to have greater confidence in our ability to cope when activating events arise.

Gratitude

Gratitude relates to the concept of positive cognitive restructuring, as it is a proactive coping mechanism that allows us to reframe our struggles. Gratitude involves a life orientation to the positive in the world and has been shown to lead to increased social support and well-being.[20] Gratitude at work can also reduce burnout[21] and is tied to increased resilience.[22] One of the easiest ways to practice gratitude in our daily lives is to keep a gratitude journal (see Box 10.1). The simple act of writing down what you are thankful for allows for reflection on the positive aspects of life and can lead to a reframing of negative thought patterns. In a seminal study by Robert Emmons and colleagues, researchers found that people who kept gratitude lists were more likely to make progress in personal goals, be more optimistic, exercise more regularly, and feel better about their lives as a whole.[23]

Meditation and mindfulness

Meditation and mindfulness are two coping strategies that have been widely adopted. Meditation has been practiced for thousands of years and

---

Box 10.1 Making the Most Out of a Gratitude Journal

- Each day, write down three to five things that you are thankful for.
- Relive the situations in your memory and reflect: Why did the situation take place? What was right about it? How did you react to it?
- Now, think about a negative experience. What was your emotional response? What thoughts or actions helped improve your mood?
- Over time, this exercise should help you to understand your negative thought patterns and allow you to refocus your mental energy toward positive thinking.

originated as a religious tool to deepen understanding of the spiritual forces of life. These days, meditation is commonly used as a tool for relaxation and stress reduction. The use of meditation continues to increase in the United States, with 4.1 percent of adults reporting that they meditated in 2012, growing to 14.2 percent in 2017.[24] Meditation may decrease stress by affecting the autonomic nervous system and mitigating the stress response.[25] Functional magnetic resonance imaging studies indicate that meditation activates neural structures involved in attention (frontal and parietal cortex) and arousal/autonomic control (pregenual anterior cingulate, amygdala, midbrain, and hypothalamus).[26] The *relaxation response* associated with meditation has been shown to lower heart rates, blood pressure, and oxygen consumption and alleviate symptoms of many conditions.[27] Meditation has also been shown to lead to structural changes in the brain. A study of experienced daily meditators found that meditation is associated with increased cortical thickness.[28]

It is clear that meditation produces many benefits for well-being. However, many people choose not to meditate because of misconceptions about the practice.[29] They may believe that they do not have enough time to meditate, or that one must be spiritual to meditate, or that meditation is too boring or too difficult. Although becoming proficient in meditation requires practice like any other skill, it can be as simple as closing your eyes and focusing on your breathing for one minute or taking a walk and paying increased attention to your senses and surroundings. There is not a single, correct way to practice meditation, and you should seek to find a strategy that works for you. However, taking just a few minutes out of your day to meditate may help tremendously to cope with stress.

Those who may be put off by the spiritual connotations of meditation may be more willing to engage in mindfulness, as it was developed entirely as a secular practice. Mindfulness refers to the practice of maintaining a state of awareness of one's thoughts, emotions, or experience. Many of the same strategies used in meditation are incorporated to develop mindfulness, such as mindfulness meditation, body awareness, and exploration of patterns of thinking.

Jon Kabat-Zinn developed mindfulness-based stress reduction (MBSR) to empower individuals to develop mindfulness and respond consciously to external stressors rather than automatically.[30] The efficacy of MBSR in reducing stress has been well documented,[31] and MBSR programs have been adopted in many medical schools and residency programs.[32] In addition, MBSR may lead to permanent improvements to well-being by changing the structure of the brain. Mindfulness practice, like meditation, has been shown to cause changes in the gray matter composition of the hippocampus and amygdala, limbic-system structures implicated in emotional regulation as well as memory and learning.[33,34] Also, MBSR has been shown to increase self-compassion, meaning that it can contribute to the development of a growth mindset that is inherently more resilient to stress.[35]

Social support systems

As discussed in Chapter 3, one of the main determinants of personal happiness is the quality of one's relationships. Social support can serve as a valuable coping strategy by buffering the effects of stress and by making harmful events seem less consequential.[36] Interestingly, social support may also help increase feelings of autonomy and enhance self-esteem. Taking the time and effort to cultivate your relationships may be one of the most valuable investments for your well-being. It also might not be as difficult as you think. You don't have to formalize your social support network; a quick coffee break with a coworker, a virtual meeting or a phone call with a close friend, or volunteer work for something you are passionate about are all ways to develop and maintain meaningful relationships (see Box 10.2).

An effective social support system should include relationships in both the professional and personal spheres. Social support in the professional

---

Box 10.2 Ideas for Cultivating your Social Support Network

- Stay connected with friends and family using online social media networks.
- Take a class and meet others who share your interests.
- Adopt a pet.
- Re-evaluate relationships and let go of toxic ones.
- Plan meetings with colleagues, for example a monthly dinner.

setting may help increase feelings of engagement and activation, allowing for one to find meaning in the workplace. As we mentioned in Chapter 8 of this volume, effective teams can help protect against burnout. Building peer support systems represents a shift from a culture of silence to a culture of sharing, acceptance, and psychological safety.[37] Social support in the personal setting is important for decompression or the ability to separate oneself from the stresses of work. Regardless of the setting, cultivating social networks is an active process that requires effort. Relationships are a two-way street and require nurturing. Nevertheless, the benefits are likely to be worth the effort.

Maladaptive coping

Maladaptive or noncoping strategies reduce symptoms while maintaining or strengthening the stressor. These strategies may sometimes be effective temporarily but are not effective in the long-term. Maladaptive coping strategies include anxious avoidance, denial, dissociation, and even substance use. Anxious avoidance is one of the most commonly employed maladaptive coping strategies: simply avoiding situations that make one anxious. This is a double-edged sword. While being able to say "no" to commitments that you cannot handle is a valuable skill, seeking to avoid all stressful situations is unfeasible and also tends to exacerbate stress in the long run.[38]

A national survey of substance use disorders among physicians found that 12.9 percent of male physicians and 21.4 percent of female physicians met diagnostic criteria for alcohol abuse or dependence.[39] Furthermore, physicians have been found to have higher rates of prescription drug abuse when compared to the general population.[40] Two of the major reasons cited by physicians for substance use were to manage emotional/psychiatric distress and to manage stressful situations, suggesting that substance use is a common maladaptive coping strategy used by the physician population.[41] Substance use by physicians has been shown to be associated with burnout, depression, suicidal ideation, and increased medical errors, and it is a major issue in healthcare (see Chapter 12 of this volume). Encouraging physicians to engage in healthy coping strategies is tied to education and training. Medical education programs ought to promote healthy coping strategies and provide the opportunities to learn and practice them.

Digital resources for stress management

There is a growing base of mobile health technologies and online programs for stress management. There are now at least 10,000 smartphone apps alone that target mental health.[42] Many of these are useful and effective. Headspace, a meditation and sleep mobile app, has been shown to increase positive affect and mindfulness in medical residents.[43] The American Medical Association has partnered with Headspace so that all members can receive a free two-year subscription. Calm is a similar guided meditation and sleep app for stress reduction. Breathe2Relax is another commonly used stress management app that guides you through diaphragmatic breathing for relaxation. A free eight-week MBSR program called Palouse Mindfulness is available online. Given the abundance of apps for stress management available, you will likely be able to find one that works for you.

Learning to gauge the safety and effectiveness of these digital technologies may be useful not only for your own well-being but also for your patients. Patients are increasingly using these easy-to-use apps and seek recommendations for appropriate programs from their physicians.[44] It is part of our responsibility as medical professionals to stay up-to-date with potential treatment modalities, including supplemental digital applications. Further research on the effectiveness of digital resources for stress management and coping is needed, particularly as the number of resources continues to grow, but it seems that they are a highly promising way to easily cope with daily stress.

Chapter Quick Summary

- Growing evidence suggests that the well-being of physicians is being eroded in the workplace. This phenomenon has been described as burnout.
- One in two physicians suffer from burnout, and while the underlying causes are mostly systemic, we have the ability to mitigate its effects through healthy coping strategies.
- Chronic stress can lead to long-term physiological and psychological damage.

- A growth mindset and self-compassion may aid in dealing with stress.
- Coping strategies can be grouped into five main categories: positive cognitive restructuring, problem-solving, seeking support, distraction, and escape/avoidance.
- Some coping strategies may be healthier and more effective than others. Maladaptive coping strategies are typically harmful in the long run.
- Examples of coping strategies include positive cognitive restructuring using the ABC technique, practicing mindfulness and meditation, and building social support systems.
- There are a variety of digital resources available for stress management.

Resources

American Institute of Stress. "Mental Health Apps." https://www.stress.org/mental-health-apps

American Medical Association. "AMA STEPS Forward." *AMA EdHub*. https://edhub.ama-assn.org/steps-forward

American Psychiatric Association. "App Evaluation Model." *App Adviser*. https://www.psychiatry.org/psychiatrists/practice/mental-health-apps/the-app-evaluation-model

National Academy of Medicine. "Action Collaborative on Clinician Well-Being and Resilience." https://nam.edu/resources-from-the-action-collaborative-on-clinician-well-being-and-resilience/

References

1. Dyrbye, L.N., C.P. West, D. Satele, S. Boone, L. Tan, J. Sloan, and T.D. Shanafelt. "Burnout among U.S. Medical Students, Residents, and Early Career Physicians Relative to the General U.S. Population." *Acad Med* 89, no. 3 (2014): 443–451. https://doi.org/10.1097/ACM.0000000000000134
2. National Academies of Sciences, Engineering, and Medicine; National Academy of Medicine; and Committee on Systems Approaches to Improve Patient Care

by Supporting Clinician Well-Being. *Taking Action Against Clinician Burnout: A Systems Approach to Professional Well-Being.* Washington, DC: National Academies Press, 2019. http://www.ncbi.nlm.nih.gov/books/NBK552618/

3. Rosenstein, A.H. "Hospital Administration Response to Physician Stress and Burnout." *Hosp Pract* 47, no. 5 (2019): 217–220. https://doi.org/10.1080/21548331.2019.1688596

4. Selye, H. "The General Adaptation Syndrome and The Diseases of Adaptation." *J Clin Endocrinol Metab* 6, no. 2 (1946): 117–230. https://doi.org/10.1210/jcem-6-2-117

5. Yaribeygi, H., Y. Panahi, H. Sahraei, T.P. Johnston, and A. Sahebkar. "The Impact of Stress on Body Function: A Review." *EXCLI J* 16 (2017): 1057–1072. https://doi.org/10.17179/excli2017-480

6. Gianaros, P.J., J.R. Jennings, L.K. Sheu, P.J. Greer, L.H. Kuller, and K.A. Matthews. "Prospective Reports of Chronic Life Stress Predict Decreased Grey Matter Volume in the Hippocampus." *NeuroImage* 35, no. 2 (2007): 795–803. https://doi.org/10.1016/j.neuroimage.2006.10.045

7. Osório, C., T. Probert, E. Jones, A.H. Young, and I. Robbins. "Adapting to Stress: Understanding the Neurobiology of Resilience." *Behav Med* 43, no. 4 (2017): 307–322. https://doi.org/10.1080/08964289.2016.1170661

8. Nakamura, J., and M. Csikszentmihalyi. "The Concept of Flow." In *Flow and the Foundations of Positive Psychology: The Collected Works of Mihaly Csikszentmihalyi.* Edited by M. Csikszentmihalyi, 239–263. Dordrecht, The Netherlands: Springer, 2014. https://doi.org/10.1007/978-94-017-9088-8_16

9. Lazarus, R.S., and S. Folkman. *Stress, Appraisal, and Coping.* New York: Springer, 1984.

10. Dweck, C.S. *Mindset: The New Psychology of Success.* Updated ed. New York: Ballantine Books, 2007.

11. Allen, A.B., and M.R. Leary. "Self-Compassion, Stress, and Coping." *Soc Personal Psychol* 4, no. 2 (2010): 107–118. https://doi.org/10.1111/j.1751-9004.2009.00246.x

12. Schroder, H.S., M.M. Yalch, S. Dawood, C.P. Callahan, M. Brent Donnellan, and J. Moser. "Growth Mindset of Anxiety Buffers the Link between Stressful Life Events and Psychological Distress and Coping Strategies." *Per Individ Differ* 110 (2017): 23–26. https://doi.org/10.1016/j.paid.2017.01.016

13. Penley, J.A., J. Tomaka, and J.S. Wiebe. "The Association of Coping to Physical and Psychological Health Outcomes: A Meta-analytic Review." *J Behav Med* 25, no. 6 (2002): 551–603. https://doi.org/10.1023/a:1020641400589.

14. Laranjeira, C.A. "The Effects of Perceived Stress and Ways of Coping in a Sample of Portuguese Health Workers." *J Clinic Nurs* 21(11–12) (2012): 1755–1762. https://doi.org/10.1111/j.1365-2702.2011.03948.x

15. Healy, C.M., and M.F. McKay. "Nursing Stress: The Effects of Coping Strategies and Job Satisfaction in a Sample of Australian Nurses." *J Adv Nurs* 31, no. 3 (2000): 681–688. https://doi.org/10.1046/j.1365-2648.2000.01323.x

16. Rafnsson, F.D., F.H. Jonsson, and M. Windle. "Coping Strategies, Stressful Life Events, Problem Behaviors, and Depressed Affect." *Anxiety Stress Coping* 19, no. 3 (2006): 241–257. https://doi.org/10.1080/10615800600679111

17. Roth, S., and L. Cohen. "Approach, Avoidance, and Coping with Stress." *Am Psychol* 41, no. 7 (1986): 813–819. https://doi.org/10.1037/0003-066x.41.7.813

18. Skinner, E.A., K. Edge, J. Altman, and H. Sherwood. "Searching for the Structure of Coping: A Review and Critique of Category Systems for Classifying Ways of Coping." *Psychol Bull* 129, no. 2 (2003): 216–269. https://doi.org/10.1037/0033-2909.129.2.216

19. Ellis, A. *Reason and Emotion in Psychotherapy.* New York: Lyle Stuart, 1962.

20. Wood, A.M., J. Maltby, R. Gillett, P.A. Linley, and S. Joseph. "The Role of Gratitude in the Development of Social Support, Stress, and Depression: Two Longitudinal Studies." *J Res Person* 42, no. 4 (2008): 854–871. https://doi.org/10.1016/j.jrp.2007.11.003

21. Chan, D.W. "Burnout and Life Satisfaction: Does Gratitude Intervention Make a Difference among Chinese School Teachers in Hong Kong?" *Ed Psychol* 31, no. 7 (2011): 809–823. https://doi.org/10.1080/01443410.2011.608525

22. Green, J.D., J.L. Davis, A.H. Cairo, B.J. Griffin, A.M.C. Behler, and R.C. Garthe. "Relational Predictors and Correlates of Humility: An Interdependence Analysis." In *Handbook of Humility: Theory, Research, and Applications.* Edited by E.L. Worthington Jr., D.E. Davis, and J.N. Hook, 165–177. New York: Routledge, 2017.

23. Emmons, R.A., and M.E. McCullough. "Counting Blessings versus Burdens: An Experimental Investigation of Gratitude and Subjective Well-Being in Daily Life." *J Pers Soc Psychol* 84, no. 2 (2003): 377–389. https://doi.org/10.1037//0022-3514.84.2.377

24. Clarke, T.C., P.M. Barnes, L.I. Black, B.J. Stussman, and R.L. Nahin. "Use of Yoga, Meditation, and Chiropractors among U.S. Adults Aged 18 and Over." *NCHS Data Brief* 325 (2018): 1–8.

25. Gamaiunova, L., P.-Y. Brandt, G. Bondolfi, and M. Kliegel. "Exploration of Psychological Mechanisms of the Reduced Stress Response in Long-Term

Meditation Practitioners." *Psychoneuroendocrinology* 104 (2019): 143–151. https://doi.org/10.1016/j.psyneuen.2019.02.026

26. Lazar, S.W., G. Bush, R.L. Gollub, G.L. Fricchione, G. Khalsa, and H. Benson. "Functional Brain Mapping of the Relaxation Response and Meditation." *Neuroreport* 11, no. 7 (2000): 1581–1585.

27. Galvin, J.A., H. Benson, G.R. Deckro, G.L. Fricchione, and J.A. Dusek. "The Relaxation Response: Reducing Stress and Improving Cognition in Healthy Aging Adults." *Complement Ther Clin Pract* 12, no. 3 (2006): 186–191. https://doi.org/10.1016/j.ctcp.2006.02.004

28. Lazar, S.W., C.E. Kerr, R.H. Wasserman, J.R. Gray, D.N. Greve, M.T. Treadway, M. McGarvey, B.T. Quinn, J.A. Dusek, H. Benson, S.L. Rauch, C.I. Moore, and B. Fischl. "Meditation Experience Is Associated with Increased Cortical Thickness." *Neuroreport* 16, no. 17 (2005): 1893–1897. https://doi.org/10.1097/01.wnr.0000186598.66243.19

29. Williams, A., P. Van Ness, J. Dixon, and R. McCorkle. "Barriers to Meditation by Gender and Age among Cancer Family Caregivers." *Nurs Res* 61, no. 1 (2012): 22–27. https://doi.org/10.1097/NNR.0b013e3182337f4d

30. Kabat-Zinn, J., L. Lipworth, and R. Burney. "The Clinical Use of Mindfulness Meditation for the Self-Regulation of Chronic Pain." *J Behav Med* 8, no. 2 (1985): 163–190. https://doi.org/10.1007/BF00845519

31. Khoury, B., M. Sharma, S.E. Rush, and C. Fournier. "Mindfulness-Based Stress Reduction for Healthy Individuals: A Meta-Analysis." *J Psychosom Res* 78, no. 6 (2015): 519–528. https://doi.org/10.1016/j.jpsychores.2015.03.009

32. Barnes, N., P. Hattan, D.S. Black, and Z. Schuman-Olivier. "An Examination of Mindfulness-Based Programs in US Medical Schools." *Mindfulness* 8, no. 2 (2017): 489–494. https://doi.org/10.1007/s12671-016-0623-8.

33. Hölzel, B.K., J. Carmody, K.C. Evans, E.A. Hoge, J.A. Dusek, L. Morgan, R.K. Pitman, and S.W. Lazar. "Stress Reduction Correlates with Structural Changes in the Amygdala." *Soc Cogn Affect Neurosci* 5, no. 1 (2010): 11–17. https://doi.org/10.1093/scan/nsp034

34. Hölzel, B.K., J. Carmody, M. Vangel, C. Congleton, S.M. Yerramsetti, T. Gard, and S.W. Lazar. "Mindfulness Practice Leads to Increases in Regional Brain Gray Matter Density." *Psych Res* 191, no. 1 (2011): 36–43. https://doi.org/10.1016/j.pscychresns.2010.08.006

35. Raab, K. "Mindfulness, Self-Compassion, and Empathy Among Health Care Professionals: A Review of the Literature." *J Health Care Chaplain* 20, no. 3 (2014): 95–108. https://doi.org/10.1080/08854726.2014.913876

36. Ozbay, F., D.C. Johnson, E. Dimoulas, C.A. Morgan, D. Charney, and S. Southwick. "Social Support and Resilience to Stress." *Psychiatry (Edgmont)* 4, no. 5 (2007): 35–40.

37. AMA STEPS Forward. "Peer Support Programs for Physicians" [Course]. *AMA EdHub*. June 25, 2020. https://edhub.ama-assn.org/steps-forward/module/ 2767766

38. Dijkstra, M.T.M., and A.C. Homan. "Engaging in Rather than Disengaging from Stress: Effective Coping and Perceived Control." *Frontiers Psychol* 7 (2016). https://doi.org/10.3389/fpsyg.2016.01415

39. Oreskovich, M.R., T. Shanafelt, L.N. Dyrbye, L. Tan, W. Sotile, D. Satele, C.P. West, J. Sloan, and S. Boone. "The Prevalence of Substance Use Disorders in American Physicians." *Am J Addict* 24, no, 1 (2015): 30–38. https://doi.org/ 10.1111/ajad.12173

40. Hughes, P.H., N. Brandenburg, D.C. Baldwin, C.L. Storr, K.M. Williams, J.C. Anthony, and D.V. Sheehan. "Prevalence of Substance Use among US Physicians." *JAMA* 267, no. 17 (1992): 2333–2339.

41. Merlo, L.J., S. Singhakant, S.M. Cummings, and L. B. Cottler. "Reasons for Misuse of Prescription Medication Among Physicians Undergoing Monitoring by a Physician Health Program." *J Addict Med* 7, no. 5 (2013): 349–353. https:// doi.org/10.1097/ADM.0b013e31829da074

42. Torous, J., and L.W. Roberts. "Needed Innovation in Digital Health and Smartphone Applications for Mental Health: Transparency and Trust." *JAMA Psychiatry* 74, no. 5 (2017): 437–438. https://doi.org/10.1001/ jamapsychiatry.2017.0262

43. Wen, L., T.E. Sweeney, L. Welton, M. Trockel, and L. Katznelson. "Encouraging Mindfulness in Medical House Staff via Smartphone App: A Pilot Study." *Acad Psych* 41, no. 5 (2017): 646–650. https://doi.org/10.1007/s40596-017-0768-3

44. Sandoval, L.R., J. Torous, and M.S. Keshavan. "Smartphones for Smarter Care? Self-Management in Schizophrenia." *Amer J Psych* 174, no. 8 (2017): 725–728. https://doi.org/10.1176/appi.ajp.2017.16090990

11

Depression, Anxiety, and Physician Suicide

Physicians perform life-saving surgeries, deliver compassionate care, and conduct groundbreaking research. We follow a calling to serve others, yet it is increasingly evident that we, as a profession, have largely neglected to serve ourselves. This is evidenced by the physician burnout epidemic, which affects approximately half of all physicians (see Chapter 10 of this volume). Even more troubling are the statistics of physician mental illness and suicide. While physicians are less likely than the general population to die of illnesses such as heart disease, chronic obstructive pulmonary disease, and cancer, they are significantly more likely to die of suicide. Although the exact numbers are not known, three to four hundred physicians are estimated to die by suicide each year, enough to fill multiple medical school classes. Many of the same factors that contribute to burnout also contribute to the prevalence of mental health disorders among physicians. High levels of professional stress, compounded with diminished autonomy and decreased job satisfaction, are often-cited factors for both depression and suicidality among physicians, although the etiologies may be different.

While suicide represents the convergence of many different risk factors, the most common one is untreated or improperly managed mental health conditions.[1] Physicians possess a deeper health knowledge and have greater access to care than the general population, but they often do not seek out professional help for mental health issues. This also has many causes, but perhaps most significant is the stigma associated with mental illness within the profession. Stigmatization occurs at many levels: self, colleagues, hospitals/ medical system, and licensing boards. For example, striving for perfection— which is a common trait among physicians—may cause cognitive dissonance in physicians and trainees when suffering with mental health disorders, potentially leading them to ignore or minimize the problem. Colleagues may be unwilling to discuss mental health issues. Hospital systems may discriminate against or stereotype physicians who bring up these issues. Many licensing boards continue to ask physicians to disclose their history of treatment for mental health illnesses, even if they have successfully received treatment. And while depression and other mental health conditions begin early—with the prevalence of depression and depressive symptoms in both medical school students[2] and residents[3] estimated to be around 30 percent—the stigma against seeking help also begins early. Only 15.7 percent of medical students who screened positive for depression reported seeking psychiatric treatment.[2] In addition, the majority of medical students who self-reported mental illness stated that they would not disclose this information in a license application.[4]

Physicians suffer from a range of mental health disorders at rates similar to or greater than the general population, including depression and substance use disorders (see Chapter 12 of this volume). Physicians are also likely to suffer from other psychiatric disorders prevalent within the general population, including bipolar disorders, anxiety disorders, obsessive-compulsive disorder, and eating disorders, but little research has been done regarding their prevalence and impact. Improving physician mental health begins with erasing the stigma around it and bringing awareness to it. As medical professionals, we have a mandate to care for ourselves.

Addressing mental health illnesses in physicians is also important for improving the health outcomes of patients. Depressed residents were found to make 6.2 times as many medication errors compared to their nondepressed counterparts.[5] Depression and anxiety have also been linked to breakdowns in physician–patient relationships.[6] It is evident that physician mental illnesses are a public health concern that need to be addressed, for the well-being of physicians and their patients alike.

Depressive disorders

Depressive disorders represent one of the most common categories of psychiatric disorders. Depressive disorders are heterogeneous, ranging from acute and severe disorders such as major depressive disorder to more chronic, low-grade disorders such as dysthymia. They may be caused by other underlying conditions, such as substance use or hormonal changes. It is therefore difficult to make broad statements about them. Nevertheless, all depressive disorders have a common component of a sad, empty, or irritable mood, accompanied by somatic and cognitive changes that affect function.[7]

The most commonly diagnosed depressive disorder is major depressive disorder (MDD), and it is likely that most depressed physicians suffer from MDD. While many of the symptoms of MDD are similar to those of burnout, burnout is a syndrome that represents a breakdown in the relationship between people and their work, whereas depression is a chronic disease that may have multifactorial causes. Although those who suffer from burnout may be at higher risk of depression, and vice versa, it is important to make the distinction between the two concepts.

Depression is also distinct from sadness. While sadness is a primary symptom of depression, it is a normal emotion that is typically elicited by a specific situation, person, or event: a trigger. Feelings of sadness in depression typically do not require a trigger and are persistent. When feelings of sadness are persistent over a period of two years, the condition may be diagnosed as dysthymia, a form of chronic depression. It is important to note that self-harm and suicidal ideations are typically not associated with nondepressive sadness but are common symptoms of MDD.

Physician depression

Medical students have similar rates of depression to the general population when they enter medical school. However, as they continue their education and training, depression rates rise. Approximately one-fourth of first- and second-year medical students surveyed were depressed, according to a study at University of California San Francisco.[8] As students progress through their education and training, rates of depression tend to increase even further, to around 30 percent in residency.[9] Many of the underlying causes are the same as for burnout (see Chapter 10 of this volume). Long work hours, high levels of personal and professional stress, as well as decreased autonomy and engagement are some of the commonly cited factors for both depression and burnout.[10]

After completing residency, the risk of depression persists. Although research suggests that attending physicians suffer from lower rates of depression as compared to residents, their prevalence of depression is still greater than that of the general population.[11] Feelings of hopelessness and worthlessness associated with depression frequently lead to declines in professional performance, affecting patient outcomes. Personal and professional relationships may be harmed over time, further damaging one's ability to cope with stress. Furthermore, physicians suffering from depression may seek to leave the profession, incurring additional costs to the profession.[12]

The good news is that preventative strategies that target depression are likely to be effective. A study of high-risk groups found that preventative interventions reduced onset of depression by as much as 25 to 50 percent.[13] Furthermore, although physicians may be wary to begin taking prophylactic medication, psychological interventions alone, primarily in the form of cognitive-behavioral therapy, have been shown to be efficacious for preventing the incidence of depression.[14] Physicians who seek out psychiatric help are likely to experience improvement in their depressive symptoms.

Physician suicide

Untreated depression among physicians is particularly worrying because of the increased risk for suicide. The data suggest that physicians are more likely to commit suicide compared to the general population. In a survey of 7,905 surgeons in the United States, 6.3 percent reported suicidal ideation within the past year.[15] Male physicians have suicide rates up to 40 percent higher than their general population cohort, and female physicians have suicide rates up to 130 percent higher.[16] These discrepancies may be due to knowledge regarding human biology and access to medications that comes with being a physician. In fact, the second most common method of suicide among physicians is by poisoning,[17] whereas suicide by poisoning is unlikely to be successful among the general population.[18] The fact that physicians are generally more successful in their suicide attempts is highly concerning, because the decision to commit suicide is often impulsive and most who fail regret their decision.[19] Consider the story in Box 11.1 of one doctor who attempted suicide.

Stories such as Michael's are unfortunately not uncommon in the medical profession. However, physician suicide is not getting the attention it deserves. Although it is estimated that up to 400 physicians die from suicide every year, those surrounding the problem often choose not to address it. A culture

Box 11.1 Case Study on Physician Suicide

As an emergency room physician, Michael faced difficult decisions and crisis situations every day; however, it was a casual decision he made that almost ended his life. When a young girl came in with the flu, he followed standard procedures, performed a few treatments, and then allowed her to go home with the proper warnings. She came back, a few days later, in respiratory arrest and ended up on life support. The family was vocal about their disdain for the physician and would not withdraw care. A few days later, the physician learned in his review that he was to be terminated due to this case and a few other minor incidents, despite support and empathy from his employers. Initially distraught, he talked through the issue with his wife, determined he could return to work at a previous job, and he moved on, returning to work that night.

Unfortunately, practicing medicine and experiencing the constant trauma associated with it can have a significant effect on the mental health of those who choose it as a career. This physician felt the weight of heart-wrenching cases that had made their way through his emergency room in the past: a woman shot in a domestic abuse case; or a child beaten to death for acting out. He had gone on a rescue-and-recovery trip abroad and experienced dead bodies melting in the heat. But this last girl who he failed to save just happened to push him over the edge. When he came home from work early the next morning, he cried himself to sleep, woke up still feeling sad, and decided to end his life.

Note that Michael loved his wife and had a pleasant personal life. Despite his support system and the fact that most aspects of his life were intact, the memory of past anguish was enough to set off this chain of events. He drove into the mountains and took a handful of pills, but he was pulled over by the police and taken to the hospital. His life was saved, and he now expresses great joy that he did not die that day. Nevertheless, he is not sure if he will ever return to the ER to work as a physician.

of silence exists. Physician obituaries often claim that death occurred in an accident or give no cause of death. At funerals, family members and friends talk about the achievements and wonderful qualities of the deceased but do not mention their struggles with their work or their depression. Colleagues choose not to discuss the suicide and return to seeing patients, sometimes while feeling guilt that they could not or did not prevent the death. The institutions responsible for the circumstances in which these doctors toil wish to ignore the problem. But this silence only puts more physicians in jeopardy. It maintains the stigma surrounding the discussion of suicide and discourages those in need from seeking help. It is challenging but necessary for doctors to speak up about suicide and depression. Sometimes the realization that they are not alone is all it takes to get a suicidal physician on the path to recovery.

Anxiety disorders

Anxiety disorders have been less well-studied than depression in physicians. However, evidence suggests that they are also prevalent within the physician population. The challenges of medical training and practice—compounded with the same common character traits such as neuroticism and perfectionism that are associated with depression—likely lead to high rates of anxiety within the physician population. Indeed, one review of medical students in the United States and Canada revealed higher incidence of anxiety as compared to the general population.[20] A deeper understanding of anxiety disorders among physicians is necessary and awaits further research. However, it seems likely that improving the professional culture to emphasize wellness and self-care will have benefits for reducing anxiety disorders among physicians.

A major barrier to care: the stigma against mental health illnesses

The stigma against mental health disorders is unfortunately one of the main factors preventing those struggling from getting the help they need. According to Kristin Raj, stigma about mental illness is pervasive in medicine and may manifest at different levels: self, colleagues, hospitals/medical systems, and licensing boards.[21]

The stigma often begins with the individual themselves. Neuroticism, self-criticism, and perfectionism are traits that are common among physicians that may lead to self-stigmatization.[22] Physicians who suffer from mental health disorders may view themselves as incapable or weak, instead of suffering from an illness that requires treatment. Colleagues may be afraid to broach the topic of mental health and fail to refer their peers to professional help until it is too late. Hospitals/medical systems are likely to label the actions of physicians suffering from mental health issues as "unprofessional" and seek out punitive action instead of taking more nuanced action that supports the well-being of the physician. Lastly, licensing boards may discriminate against physicians who disclose prior psychiatric history, meaning that mental health disorders among physicians often go undiagnosed and untreated. The Americans with Disabilities Act currently recommends that employers assess only current functional impairment; however, many state licensing boards continue to ask about prior psychiatric history.[23] The American Psychiatric Association also states that when assessing for current impairment, the presence of prior psychiatric history is not relevant, indicating that this practice is inappropriate and stigmatizing.[24] These stigmatizing forces only serve to increase the prevalence of physicians who suffer from undiagnosed and untreated mental health conditions, which only increases the risk of damage to both physician and patient well-being.

The culture of silence also creates blurred lines regarding what is and is not appropriate regarding physicians who are suffering from mental illness. Are we to report colleagues suffering from depression? Will we be suspended if we are found out to be practicing with a diagnosed mental illness? What are the laws, and are there legal precedents? Many of these questions go unanswered because physicians are wary to broach the topic of mental health due to stigma.

Although many policies are state- and institution-specific, whenever patient safety may be potentially harmed, physicians have an ethical duty as professionals to report. Often it is best to report anonymously to a physician health program (see Chapter 12 of this volume) rather than the state medical board. If physicians are reported to the state medical board before involvement with a physician health program, they may be subject to a formal disciplinary action and at risk of losing their license. It is also important to remember that not all mental health conditions prevent physicians from practicing without impairment. Just because you or a colleague are suffering from anxiety or depression does not mean that you are automatically impaired and at risk of damaging patient safety. This is, of course, a judgment call. If you are suffering from mental health illness without functional impairment, seek out professional help in a way that is confidential. If you suspect that a colleague may be suffering from a mental health disorder that is not causing functional impairment, keep an eye out, and be sure to intervene in a timely manner to address the issue before it is too late. As difficult as it may be, letting your colleague know that you are there to support them, confidentially referring them to a mental health professional may be an important step on the path to recovery.

According to ADA guidelines, physicians who suffer from mental health illness may not be discriminated against. However, yet again the policies are blurry. The ADA states that to be protected, at least one of three requirements must be satisfied: a physical or mental impairment that prevents you from performing a major life activity, a medical history of suffering from a physical or mental ailment, or the perception that you suffer from a physical or mental impairment. Then the physician must prove that their condition hinders their work performance. Physicians will likely not document that their mental health condition affects their performance, because then they are at risk for disciplinary action or suspension of licensure. Unfortunately, the current guidelines regarding mental health also serve to propagate stigma.

It is undoubtedly a difficult situation for physicians suffering from mental health disorders, and widespread action is needed to change the attitudes and beliefs about mental health within the profession. Nevertheless, physicians, at least for now, ought to at least learn the specific guidelines that they must abide by. Much of this information can be found in state board documents and in institutional policies.

Improving physician mental health

The first step to improving mental health within the physician population is to learn to recognize the signs of mental health illness. There are some telltale signs that you can look out for, both for yourself and your colleagues (see Box 11.2).

Although recognizing the symptoms of mental health illnesses in ourselves and our colleagues is a good first step, a profession-wide change in attitudes about mental health is needed. This requires actions at many different levels. Individually, physicians can reflect on their own thoughts and

---

Box 11.2 Common Signs of Mental Health Conditions

- Hopeless outlook
- Changes in eating or sleeping habits
- Persistent irritability
- Overwhelming fatigue
- Loss of interest
- Difficulty concentrating
- Extreme mood changes
- Detachment from reality (delusions) and paranoia

---

attitudes that may be leading to the propagation of stigma against mental health. Such thoughts could be as benign as "I should be able to push through this; I've made it this far" or "We are all working hard; I shouldn't complain." Recognizing that these thoughts are contributing to stigmatization for yourself and for your colleagues is a valuable step in promoting a culture of mental health. Furthermore, identifying specific resources for mental health for oneself or for colleagues may also be helpful.

At the organizational level, hospitals may seek to institute widespread, confidential depression and mental health screenings for physicians. This is a strategy that has been adopted by a few organizations, such as the University of California San Diego through its Healer Education Assessment and Referral (HEAR) program, which has been shown to be effective.[25] This may be a model to emulate, although organizations should be careful to ensure that screenings and referrals are done in a confidential manner. In-house mental health providers may also be effective for physicians who cite that lack of time is a barrier to accessing proper care. Administrators should also seek to take a nuanced approach that promotes health of providers rather than punishment for "unprofessional" behaviors that stem from mental health conditions.

Reform is also necessary at the level of state licensing boards. In 2017, 84 percent of state licensing forms contained questions about mental health.[26] Unlike questions regarding physical health, these questions tend to include treatment history, with only 53 percent of the applications focusing on functional impairment. However, the American Medical Association recommends that state boards "evaluate a physician's mental and physical health similarly, ensuring that a previously diagnosed mental health illness is not automatically considered as a current impairment to practice."[27] A push to change the licensing board questions to normalize mental health and reduce the stigma associated with it will likely be a valuable step for preserving physician mental health. Additionally, improved education on effective coping strategies to deal with stress (see Chapter 10 of this volume) as well as on lifestyle interventions that improve mental health (see Chapters 3 and 9 of this volume) is also likely to be a part of the solution.

Chapter Quick Summary

- Physicians suffer from mental health issues, particularly depression, at higher rates than the general population, due to many of the same factors that contribute to burnout.
- There is a stigma within the profession that prevents physicians suffering from psychiatric disorders from getting the help they need.
- Stigma can result from self, from colleagues, from hospitals/medical systems, and from licensing boards.
- Approximately 300 to 400 physicians are estimated to die from suicide each year, and untreated mental health conditions are a significant risk factor.
- The stigma around mental illness often blurs the lines of appropriate action regarding mental health.
- Action at individual, institutional, and organizational levels is necessary to combat the stigma of mental illness and ensure that physicians are able to receive the mental healthcare that they need.

Resources

Accreditation Council for Graduate Medicine Education. "Back to Bedside Project Highlights." https://www.acgme.org/Residents-and-Fellows/Back-to-Bedside/Back-to-Bedside-Project-Highlights

American Foundation for Suicide Prevention. "Partners." https://afsp.org/partners

American Foundation for Suicide Prevention. "Suicide Prevention Resources." https://afsp.org/suicide-prevention-resources#crisis-services

American Hospital Association. "The Physician Well-Being Playbook." https://www.aha.org/physicians/well-playbook

American Psychiatric Organization. "Well-Being Resources." https://www.psychiatry.org/psychiatrists/practice/well-being-and-burnout/well-being-resources

Bhatt, J., and J. Reed. "Suicide Prevention Resources Available to Help Physicians." *American Hospital Association.* September 17, 2019. https://www.aha.org/news/insights-and-analysis/2019-09-17-suicide-prevention-resources-available-help-physicians

E-Couch. [Home page]. https://ecouch.com.au/

Massachusetts General Hospital. "Guide to Mental Health Resources for COVID-19." https://www.massgeneral.org/psychiatry/guide-to-mental-health-resources/?fbclid=IwAR2vo1TZVRS0FMYI_vpWjCiiyDhZPxPNdXNlo0JP50Ajp3YFLpMeSingAX0

Neff, K. "Mindful Self-Compassion." 2020. https://self-compassion.org/the-program/

Suicide Prevention Lifeline. [Home page]. https://suicidepreventionlifeline.org/

Suicide Prevention Resource Center. "Resources and Programs." http://www.sprc.org/resources-programs

U.S. Department of Veteran Affairs. "PTSD: National Center for PTSD: Apps, Videos and More." https://www.ptsd.va.gov/appvid/index.asp

References

1. Brådvik, L. "Suicide Risk and Mental Disorders." *Int J Environ Res Public Health* 15, no. 9 (2018). https://doi.org/10.3390/ijerph15092028

2. Rotenstein, L.S., M.A. Ramos, M. Torre, J.B. Segal, M.J. Peluso, C. Guille, S. Sen, and D.A. Mata. "Prevalence of Depression, Depressive Symptoms, and Suicidal Ideation Among Medical Students." *JAMA* 316, no. 21 (2016): 2214–2236. https://doi.org/10.1001/jama.2016.17324

3. Mata, D.A., M.A. Ramos, N. Bansal, R. Khan, C. Guille, E. Di Angelantonio, and S. Sen. "Prevalence of Depression and Depressive Symptoms Among Resident Physicians: A Systematic Review and Meta-Analysis." *JAMA* 314, no. 22 (2015): 2373–2383. https://doi.org/10.1001/jama.2015.15845

4. Fletcher, I., M. Castle, A. Scarpa, O. Myers, and E. Lawrence. "An Exploration of Medical Student Attitudes towards Disclosure of Mental Illness." *Med Educ Online* 25, no. 1 (2020). https://doi.org/10.1080/10872981.2020.1727713

5. Fahrenkopf, A.M., T.C. Sectish, L.K. Barger, P.J. Sharek, D. Lewin, V.W. Chiang, S. Edwards, B.L. Wiedermann, and C.P. Landrigan. "Rates of Medication Errors among Depressed and Burnt out Residents: Prospective Cohort Study." *BMJ (Clinical Research Ed)* 336, no. 7642 (2008): 488–491. https://doi.org/10.1136/bmj.39469.763218.BE

6. Firth-Cozens, J. "Individual and Organizational Predictors of Depression in General Practitioners." *Br J Gen Pract* 48, no. 435 (1998):1647–1651.

7. American Psychiatric Association. *Diagnostic and Statistical Manual of Mental Disorders.* 5th ed. Arlington, VA: American Psychiatric Association, 2013.

8. Givens, J.L., and J. Tjia. "Depressed Medical Students' Use of Mental Health Services and Barriers to Use." *Acad Med* 77, no. 9 (2002): 918–921. https://doi.org/10.1097/00001888-200209000-00024

9. Mata, D.A. et al. "Prevalence of Depression and Depressive Symptoms Among Resident Physicians." JAMA 314, no. 22 (2015): 2373–2383.

10. Tomioka, K., N. Morita, K. Saeki, N. Okamoto, and N. Kurumatani. "Working Hours, Occupational Stress and Depression among Physicians." *Occup Med* 61, no. 3 (May 1, 2011): 163–70. https://doi.org/10.1093/occmed/kqr004

11. Schernhammer, E.S., and G.A. Colditz. "Suicide Rates among Physicians: A Quantitative and Gender Assessment (Meta-Analysis)." *Am J Psychiatr* 161, no. 12 (2004): 2295–2302. https://doi.org/10.1176/appi.ajp.161.12.2295

12. Degen, C., J. Li, and P. Angerer. "Physicians' Intention to Leave Direct Patient Care: An Integrative Review." *Hum Resour Health* 13 (2015). https://doi.org/10.1186/s12960-015-0068-5

13. Beekman, A.T.F., F. Smit, M.L. Stek, C.F. Reynolds, and P.C. Cuijpers. "Preventing Depression in High-Risk Groups." *Curr Opin Psychiatr* 23, no. 1 (2010): 8–11. https://doi.org/10.1097/YCO.0b013e328333e17f

14. Hetrick, S.E., G.R. Cox, K.G. Witt, J.J. Bir, and S.N. Merry. "Cognitive Behavioural Therapy (CBT), Third-wave CBT and Interpersonal Therapy (IPT) Based Interventions for Preventing Depression in Children and Adolescents." *Cochrane Database of Syst Rev* 8 (2016): CD003380. https://doi.org/10.1002/14651858.CD003380.pub4

15. Shanafelt, T.D., C.M. Balch, L. Dyrbye, G. Bechamps, T. Russell, D. Satele, T. Rummans, K. Swartz, P.J. Novotny, J. Sloan, and M.R. Oreskovich, "Special

Report: Suicidal Ideation Among American Surgeons." *AMA Arch Surg* 146, no. 1 (2011): 54–62. https://doi.org/10.1001/archsurg.2010.292

16. Schernhammer, E. "Taking Their Own Lives—The High Rate of Physician Suicide." *New Engl J Med* 352, no. 24 (June 16, 2005): 2473–2476. https://doi.org/10.1056/NEJMp058014

17. Gold, K.J., A. Sen, and T.L. Schwenk. "Details on Suicide among US Physicians: Data from the National Violent Death Reporting System." *Gen Hosp Psychiatr* 35, no. 1 (2013): 45–49. https://doi.org/10.1016/j.genhosppsych.2012.08.005

18. Spicer, R.S., and T.R. Miller. "Suicide Acts in 8 States: Incidence and Case Fatality Rates by Demographics and Method." *Am J Pub Health* 90, no. 12 (2000): 1885–1891.

19. Dombrovski, A.Y., and M.N. Hallquist. "The Decision Neuroscience Perspective on Suicidal Behavior: Evidence and Hypotheses." *Curr Opin Psychiatr* 30, no. 1 (2017): 7–14. https://doi.org/10.1097/YCO.0000000000000297

20. Dyrbye, L.N., M.R. Thomas, and T.D. Shanafelt. "Systematic Review of Depression, Anxiety, and Other Indicators of Psychological Distress among U.S. and Canadian Medical Students." *Acad Med* 81, no. 4 (April 2006): 354–373. https://doi.org/10.1097/00001888-200604000-00009

21. Raj, K.S. Mental Illness. In *The Art and Science of Physician Wellbeing: A Handbook for Physicians and Trainees.* Edited by L.W. Roberts and M. Trockel, 139–152. Cham, Switzerland: Springer Nature, 2019. https://doi.org/10.1007/978-3-319-42135-3

22. Vaillant, G.E., N.C. Sobowale, and C. McArthur. "Some Psychologic Vulnerabilities of Physicians." *New Engl J Med* 287, no. 8 (1972): 372–375. https://doi.org/10.1056/NEJM197208242870802

23. Jones, J.T.R., C.S. North, S. Vogel-Scibilia, M.F. Myers, and R.R. Owen. "Medical Licensure Questions About Mental Illness and Compliance with the Americans With Disabilities Act." *JAAPL Online* 46, no. 4 (2018): 458–471. https://doi.org/10.29158/JAAPL.003789-18

24. Boyd, J.E., B. Graunke, F.J. Frese, J.T.R. Jones, J.W. Adkins, and R. Bassman. "State Psychology Licensure Questions about Mental Illness and Compliance with the Americans with Disabilities Act." *Am J Orthopsychiat* 86, no. 6 (2016): 620–631. https://doi.org/10.1037/ort0000177

25. Norcross, W.A., C. Moutier, M. Tiamson-Kassab, P. Jong, J.E. Davidson, K.C. Lee, I.G. Newton, N.S. Downs, and S. Zisook. "Update on the UC San Diego

Healer Education Assessment and Referral (HEAR) Program." *J Med Regul* 104, no. 2 (2018): 17–26. https://doi.org/10.30770/2572-1852-104.2.17

26. Gold, K.J., E.R. Shih, E.B. Goldman, and T.L. Schwenk. "Do US Medical Licensing Applications Treat Mental and Physical Illness Equivalently?" *Fam Med* 49, no. 6 (2017): 464–467.

27. American Medical Association. "AMA Adopts Policy to Improve Physician Access to Mental Health Care." June 24, 2017. https://www.ama-assn.org/ama-adopts-policy-improve-physician-access-mental-health-care

12
Substance Use Disorders and the Impaired Physician

As compared to the general population, physicians suffer from most diseases at lower rates, likely due to knowledge of medicine and incorporation of healthy lifestyle behaviors.[1] However, while the exact statistics are unknown and difficult to accurately study, the prevalence of substance use disorders (SUDs) within the physician population has been estimated to be equal to or greater than the general population. Ten to fifteen percent of physicians are estimated to develop a SUD during their careers.[2] Additionally, while physicians are less likely to abuse illicit drugs than the general population, they are more likely to abuse alcohol and prescription drugs such as opioids and benzodiazepines (see Box 12.1).[3] Physicians with untreated substance abuse problems have mortality rates estimated to be greater than 15 percent.[4] Furthermore, it is likely that these numbers are low due to the sensitive nature of physician impairment, which leads to difficulties in accurate data collection. It seems likely that poor quality data and stigma around SUDs leads to underreporting. These statistics are worrying, because SUDs not only jeopardize the well-being of the physician but also the health of patients. Indeed, alcohol use disorders in physicians have been shown to not only be associated with burnout, depression, and suicidal ideation but also with increased incidence of recent medical errors.[5]

Substance use is by no means a modern phenomenon in medicine. Sigmund Freud, at one time a renowned physician, abused and was dependent on cocaine and tobacco.[9] William Halsted, often referred to as the Father of Modern Surgery, first became addicted to cocaine, one of the anesthetics that he was testing for use in surgery, and then to morphine, which was first introduced to him as a way to break his cocaine addiction.

We have known that substance use is a problem in the medical profession for a long time. Why, then, have we failed to address it? SUDs are complex, and treating them is not as simple as prescribing a medication or performing a

Box 12.1 Substance Use Disorders in Physicians

- Alcohol is the most commonly used substance by physicians, and opioids and stimulants are the next most common.[6]
- Recreational drugs, such as marijuana or cocaine, are used less by physicians than the general population.
- Female physicians are at higher risk for SUDs[5] and have shorter time to first relapse after achieving sobriety.[7]
- Emergency medicine, psychiatry, and anesthesiology are three times as likely as other specialties to use controlled substances.[8]
- Emergency room doctors used the recreational drugs marijuana and cocaine much more than the general physician population.
- Psychiatrists used benzodiazepines more than twice as much as physicians in other specialties.
- Anesthesiologists appear to use major opioids more than their nonanesthesiologist counterparts.

procedure. SUDs may differ in severity. The fifth edition of the *Diagnostic and Statistical Manual of Mental Disorders* provides three severity specifiers: mild; moderate; and severe. Severe SUDs are also known as addictive disorders. Addiction "involves functional changes to brain circuits involved in reward, stress, and self-control" and may have effects that last long after cessation.[10] On the other hand, some SUDs may not lead to functional impairment.

Those who suffer from SUDs may avoid seeking treatment, especially if they believe that they have a lot to lose from the rehabilitation process. Also, the medical community may be hesitant to address SUDs and often fails to provide resources to assist doctors who are suffering or colleagues who wish to report. The stigma around mental health conditions (see Chapter 11 of this volume) and SUDs prevents suffering physicians from getting the help they need, putting their health and the health of their patients at risk. Furthermore, a lack of education on addiction, compounded with an ingrained professional culture of perfectionism and invincibility, serve as risk factors for SUDs in physicians.

Fortunately, the profession has begun to take steps in the right direction. In many institutions, ombuds have been established as impartial, confidential, independent, and informal third-party members who may help refer physicians to the appropriate resources.[11] Physician health programs (PHPs) have arisen as the gold standard for suffering physicians to receive treatment in a confidential manner. Seventy-eight percent of PHP participants remain substance free, with no relapse, and 71 percent of PHP participants retained their medical license and employment, at the five-year follow-up.[12] These statistics are encouraging and a good sign that PHPs work. Recently, there have been concerns expressed about oversight and regulation of PHPs.[13] Nevertheless, they represent a significant movement in the right direction for allowing suffering physicians to get the help they need.

It is evident that a profession-wide change in attitudes about mental health illnesses and SUDs is necessary to combat stigma to address the root of the problem. However, for now, as medical professionals, we can seek to learn the facts about the causes of SUDs, learn to recognize their effects, and learn the best practices for what to do if you suspect that you or a colleague is suffering from a SUD.

Epidemiology of SUDs

There are multiple causes for the prevalence of SUDs among physicians. Physicians have significantly easier access to drugs than most other professions, and substance use likely begins as a way to cope with professional stress. Indeed, in a survey of physicians who were monitored by their PHP, 69 percent said they used drugs to relieve stress and physical or emotional pain.[14] It is likely that this maladaptive coping strategy (see Chapter 10 of this volume) has roots in college, medical school, and residency. The high demands of medical education and training may lead students and trainees to set unrealistic expectations for themselves, leading to overwork and subsequent maladaptive coping. A survey of approximately 5,000 medical students from 16 medical schools found that approximately one-third of students engaged in excessive and binge drinking.[15] The relative lack of attention to SUDs in medical education may also contribute to this problem in medical trainees and also lead to inadequate preparation in diagnosing and treating SUDs as physicians.[16] In addition, after graduating medical school, perceived ability to diagnose and treat SUDs only decreases.[17] This is highly concerning and a missed opportunity for education, because SUDs are also a significant public health concern, particularly in the context of the current opioid epidemic.

Research shows that prevalence of SUDs varies by specialty. Surgeons have been shown to be more likely to use substances compared to their nonsurgeon counterparts. Five specialties—anesthesiology, emergency medicine, psychiatry, family, and internal medicine—have been found to represent the majority of physicians suffering from SUDs.[18] In particular, anesthesiologists have been found to be more likely to abuse opioids, and psychiatrists, more likely to abuse benzodiazepines. This indicates that physicians are likely to abuse drugs that they are familiar with and have access to. It is also likely that abuse of prescription medications such as opioids and benzodiazepines begin as self-treatment for stress or pain management.

Once a physician develops a SUD, the professional culture and stigma associated with mental health conditions (see Chapter 11 of this volume) prevents them from getting the help they need. Physicians are often self-reliant, independent, and perseverant. It is unlikely that they will admit to having a problem, especially if they believe they have it under control. In addition, they may believe that admission of a SUD may lead to punitive action by the hospital or even suspension of license by the state board. It is unsurprising, then, that the problem continues to persist.

Identifying impaired physicians

It is often difficult to recognize when a colleague is impaired. Impairment is defined by the American Medical Association (AMA) as when one is "unable to fulfill professional and personal responsibilities because of a psychiatric illness, alcoholism, or drug dependency"[19]; it may take many forms. It is important to recognize that impairment may result from a medical or mental illness (see Chapter 11 of this volume), from aging (see Chapter 15 of this volume), or even from stress and burnout (see Chapter 10 of this volume).[20] However, most impaired physicians suffer from a SUD.

Many physicians who suffer from SUDs are high-functioning and have developed ways to effectively hide their problem. Furthermore, symptoms of SUDs often exhibit outside of the workplace rather than inside.[21] Home life is often affected first; marital or financial problems may arise. However, work performance often remains mostly the same. Many physicians are effective at hiding their substance use in the professional setting. One study showed that

> ## Box 12.2 Signs and Symptoms of Physician Impairment in the Workplace
>
> - Frequent tardiness or absences
> - Worsening of personal hygiene
> - Increased errors in clinical judgment
> - Decreasing one's workload for no obvious reason
> - Self-prescribing or asking colleagues to prescribe substances
> - Altercations with staff or patients
> - Incorrect charting
> - Unusual rounding times
> - Increased secrecy

43 percent of opioid-using doctors had been using these drugs for more than two years before detection. Another study of physicians suffering from SUDs found that, on average, physicians displayed problematic drug use for over six years before they received treatment.[22] Often, physicians suffering with SUDs will not display any obvious symptoms. Nevertheless, there are some nonspecific signs that you can learn to recognize that may potentially suggest that there is a problem. These include behavioral or personality changes, mood swings, and atypical work behaviors (see Box 12.2).

Intervention

Prevention and early intervention are the most effective strategies to prevent the incidence and progression of SUDs. This may begin as early as medical school, for example, by questioning the use of alcohol and other substances and encouraging the adoption of healthy coping strategies and lifestyle modifications (see Chapters 9 and 10 of this volume). Creating a culture of wellness and decreasing the stresses that are placed on medical students, trainees, and physicians is also likely to be a part of the long-term solution for reducing the prevalence of SUDs.

Unfortunately, today, there are many impaired physicians continuing to practice medicine. What should you do if you believe that a colleague is suffering from a SUD that is affecting their functioning? What are your professional responsibilities? Although legal obligations may vary by state, you do have an ethical responsibility to intervene.[23] Research shows that only 67 percent of physicians will report impaired colleagues appropriately.[24] Many invested parties feel that they should not report or attempt to intervene unless they have information that proves beyond a shadow of a doubt that the physician in question is addicted. Some may believe that reporting will significantly damage their colleague's career. Others may be afraid of retaliation or think that it is not their place to report a superior. It is important to remember that a SUD is not an ethical or moral shortcoming but rather a psychiatric disorder. Intervening to report someone's SUD is about helping someone regain control of their life and career.

Depending on the progression of the SUD, it may be possible to intervene in a confidential way, without risking your colleague's license or career. Intervention is certainly difficult, and you should familiarize yourself with the best practices. Having empathy and using nonjudgmental communication is important during intervention to let colleagues know that you are advocating for their well-being. It may be helpful to recruit other people to help with the intervention. A one-on-one interaction is unlikely to produce meaningful change, as denial and avoidance are two key mechanisms used by addicts to avoid dealing with their problem. It may help to find people who know the impaired physician and have felt the impact of his or her problem. Friends and family are obvious candidates for successfully convincing an impaired physician to undergo professional evaluation and treatment. Ombuds may serve as impartial and confidential third-party members for referring colleagues and a good first step. Trusted faculty members or other confidential resources, such as the Substance Abuse and Mental Health Services Administration helpline, may also be helpful. Once you have the individual's attention, remain firm and assertive. Have a solution prepared and make a plan to directly help him or her with the first step, such as receiving a professional assessment.

Assessment and treatment

Fortunately, state law, AMA decree, and institutional understanding are beginning to catch up with this serious physician health crisis. The American Society of Addiction Medicine was formed in the 1980s to address the problem of addiction among the American public, and the American

Academy of Addiction Psychiatry was founded in 1985 to focus on the problem through the lens of psychiatry. In 1990, the Federation for State Physician Health Programs was created, and PHPs began to be incorporated into each state's physician addiction treatment toolbox. Indeed, often the best plan of action when physician impairment is suspected is to confidentially refer to a PHP, which are state agencies that seek to help physicians maintain their own health and effectiveness while protecting their rights to privacy and confidentiality.

The first PHP was established in New Jersey in 1982, as a response to a mandate by the AMA to address physician impairment in their watershed paper "The Sick Physician: Impairment by Psychiatric Disorders, Including Alcoholism and Drug Dependence."[25] By 2020, most states have established active PHPs, whose activities are coordinated by the Federation for State Physician Health Programs. PHPs serve as confidential third parties, monitoring and overseeing treatment but not treating physicians directly. Furthermore, while PHPs collaborate with state medical boards, they typically do not report monitored physicians unless they are noncompliant. The PHP approach is typically nonpunitive and therefore a good option for physicians hoping to not only fully recover but also to return to practice.

PHPs help coordinate care for physicians and provide them with social support throughout the recovery process. They advocate for their recovering physicians, helping them return to practice, and then continue to monitor them for several years. PHPs receive physicians not only through peer referral but also through self-referrals and by state medical board recommendation. Their work not only improves treatment for addicted physicians but also encourages them to seek help by providing a preferable option to remaining silent and attempting self-treatment.

Recently, some concerns about oversight and the lack of national guidelines regarding PHPs have been raised, for example, by the American College of Physicians.[26] Some PHPs have been scrutinized for inadequately protecting the rights and interests of physician participants.[27] Nevertheless, PHPs represent a step in the right direction for ensuring patient safety while providing physicians with the resources they need for recovery. As a profession, we should continue to promote nonpunitive, confidential, and standardized PHP programs in which physicians may be assured that treatment is accessible, before SUDs cause impairment and harm patient safety. The establishment of national guidelines for PHPs is now a priority for all invested parties. For example, the AMA recommends that all PHPs possess seven essential components:

1. Contingency management that includes both positive and negative consequences.
2. Random drug testing.
3. Linkage with 12-step programs and with the abstinence standard espoused by these programs.
4. Management of relapses by intensified treatment and monitoring.
5. Use of a continuing care approach.
6. Focus on lifelong recovery.
7. Protection of anonymity.[28]

Impaired physicians receive an intensity, duration, and quality of care that is rarely available to the general population. In a study of 647 physicians across 16 PHPs who were monitored for five years, 81 percent had negative urine toxicology results throughout their monitoring, and 95 percent of the 515 who completed their monitoring contract had returned to licensed work.[29] Positive outcomes for participants in PHPs are vastly greater than programs generally available to the general public, with five-year abstinence rates reported to be 75 to 90 percent.[30]

Typical treatment for recovering physicians begins with either intensive day or residential treatment to address the problem head on. This treatment is typically paired with the formation of a physician–peer support group, such as an Alcoholics Anonymous or Caduceus group. Personnel are available to advocate and plan for the return of the physician to practice after recovery, and a neuropsychiatric assessment of cognitive function can be used to determine if physicians are truly ready to return to work, both for their safety and the safety of their patients. Staff are typically available to help manage the logistical work required to get a physician back to practice, such as malpractice insurance, Drug Enforcement Agency certification, health maintenance organization relationships, and hospital medical staff liaisons. Extended treatment and continued monitoring are available to help prevent relapse and return the physician to a normal, high-performing state. Physicians have a demanding job, and it is challenging to return to normalcy after treatment, but there are a multitude of resources available to help physicians adjust. Therefore, physicians certainly should not avoid treatment because they feel that help is not available.

Having a SUD is not a moral or professional failing; SUDs are psychiatric disorders that require treatment. Physicians, whose actions have significant consequences on the health of patients, have an ethical imperative to maintain their well-being. This includes seeking out treatment for SUDs and intervening when a colleague is suspected to be impaired. Fortunately, the medical profession has begun to provide resources for impaired physicians. While further change is necessary to eliminate the stigma around mental illness and SUDs, the profession is moving in the right direction.

Chapter Quick Summary

- Approximately 10 to 15 percent of physicians will develop a substance use disorder (SUD) within their lifetimes, which is a rate greater than that of the general population.
- Substance use among physicians is not a new phenomenon in medicine; it has been documented for many decades.
- SUDs are complex and may differ in severity. They may be mild, moderate, or severe (severe SUDs are also known as addictions).
- Convenient access to substances, compounded with the stresses of the profession, may put physicians at unique risk for SUDs.
- Impaired physicians are unable to effectively fulfill professional and personal responsibilities because of a psychiatric illness, alcoholism, or drug dependency.
- Physicians have an ethical responsibility to intervene when a colleague is impaired.
- Physician health programs (PHPs) allow physicians to receive treatment in a confidential manner and help them return to practice, without risking loss of licensure.

Resources

Federation of State Medical Boards. "Report of the Special Committee on Reentry for the Ill Physician." April 2013. https://www.fsmb.org/siteassets/advocacy/policies/reentry-for-the-Ill-physician.pdf

Federation of State Physician Health Programs. [Home page]. https://www.fsphp.org/

Federation of State Physician Health Programs. "Featured Articles and Podcasts about PHPs." https://www.fsphp.org/featured-articles-and-podcasts-about-phps

Federation of State Physician Health Programs. "State Programs." https://www.fsphp.org/state-programs

Substance Abuse and Mental Health Services Administration. "National Helpline." https://www.samhsa.gov/find-help/national-helpline

References

1. Dayoub, E., and A.B. Jena. "Chronic Disease Prevalence and Healthy Lifestyle Behaviors Among US Health Care Professionals." *Mayo Clin Proc* 90, no. 12 (2015): 1659–1662. https://doi.org/10.1016/j.mayocp.2015.08.002

2. Baldisseri, M.R. "Impaired Healthcare Professional." *Crit Care Med* 35, no. 2, Suppl. (2007): S106–S116.

3. Hughes, P.H., N. Brandenburg, D.C. Baldwin, C.L. Storr, K.M. Williams, J.C. Anthony, and D.V. Sheehan. "Prevalence of Substance Use among US Physicians." *JAMA* 267, no. 17 (1992): 2333–2339.

4. Warner, D.O., K. Berge, H. Sun, A. Harman, and T. Wang. "Substance Use Disorder in Physicians after Completion of Training in Anesthesiology in the United States from 1977 to 2013." *Anesthesiology* 133, no. 2 (2020): 342–349. https://doi.org/10.1097/ALN.0000000000003310

5. Oreskovich, M.R., T. Shanafelt, L.N. Dyrbye, L. Tan, W. Sotile, D. Satele, C.P. West, J. Sloan, and S. Boone. "The Prevalence of Substance Use Disorders in American Physicians." *Am J Addict* 24, no. 1 (2015): 30–38. https://doi.org/10.1111/ajad.12173

6. Berge, K.H., M.D. Seppala, and A.M. Schipper. "Chemical Dependency and the Physician." *Mayo Clin Proc* 84, no. 7 (2009): 625–631.

7. Knight, J.R., L.T. Sanchez, L. Sherritt, L.R. Bresnahan, and J.A. Fromson. "Outcomes of a Monitoring Program for Physicians with Mental and Behavioral

Health Problems." *J Psychiatr Prac* 13, no. 1 (2007): 25–32. https://doi.org/10.1097/00131746-200701000-00004

8. Hughes, P.H., D.C. Baldwin, D.V. Sheehan, S. Conard, and C.L. Storr. "Resident Physician Substance Use, by Specialty." *Am J Psychiatr* 149, no. 10 (1992): 1348–1354. https://doi.org/10.1176/ajp.149.10.1348

9. Srivastava, A.B. "Impaired Physicians: Obliterating the Stigma." *Am J Psychiatr Resid J* 13, no. 3 (2018): 4–6. https://doi.org/10.1176/appi.ajp-rj.2018.130303.

10. National Institute on Drug Abuse. "Drug Misuse and Addiction." July 13, 2020. https://www.drugabuse.gov/publications/drugs-brains-behavior-science-addiction/drug-misuse-addiction

11. Raymond, J.R., and P.M. Layde. "Three-Year Experience of an Academic Medical Center Ombuds Office." *Acad Med* 91, no. 3 (2016): 333–337. https://doi.org/10.1097/ACM.0000000000001031

12. DuPont, R.L., A.T. McLellan, G. Carr, M. Gendel, and G.E. Skipper. "How Are Addicted Physicians Treated? A National Survey of Physician Health Programs." *J Subst Abuse Treat* 37, no. 1 (2009): 1–7. https://doi.org/10.1016/j.jsat.2009.03.010

13. Boyd, J.W., and J.R. Knight. "Ethical and Managerial Considerations Regarding State Physician Health Program." *J Addict Med* 6, no. 4 (2012): 243–46.

14. Merlo, L.J., S. Singhakant, S.M. Cummings, and L.B. Cottler. "Reasons for Misuse of Prescription Medication among Physicians Undergoing Monitoring by a Physician Health Program." *J Addict Med* 7, no. 5 (2013): 349–353. https://doi.org/10.1097/ADM.0b013e31829da074

15. Frank, E., L. Elon, T. Naimi, and R. Brewer. "Alcohol Consumption and Alcohol Counselling Behaviour among US Medical Students: Cohort Study." *BMJ* 337 (2008): a2155. https://doi.org/10.1136/bmj.a2155

16. Frank, E., L. Elon, T. Naimi, and R. Brewer. "Alcohol Consumption and Alcohol Counselling Behaviour among US Medical Students: Cohort Study." *BMJ* 337 (2008): a2155.

17. Bäck, D.K., E. Tammaro, J.K. Lim, and S.E. Wakeman. "Massachusetts Medical Students Feel Unprepared to Treat Patients with Substance Use Disorder." *J Gen Intern Med* 33, no. 3 (2018): 249–250. https://doi.org/10.1007/s11606-017-4192-x

18. Earley, P.H. "Physician Health Programs and Addiction among Physicians." In *The ASAM Essentials of Addiction Medicine.* 5th ed. Edited by R.K. Ries, D.A. Fiellin, S.C. Miller, and R. Saitz, 602–21. Philadelphia: Lippincott Williams &Wilkins, 2014.

19. "The Sick Physician. Impairment by Psychiatric Disorders, Including Alcoholism and Drug Dependence." *JAMA* 223, no. 6 (1973): 684–687.

20. Sulmasy, L.S., and T.A. Bledsoe. "American College of Physicians Ethics Manual." *Ann Intern Med* 170, no. 2, suppl. (2019): S1–S32. https://doi.org/10.7326/ M18-2160

21. Centrella, M. "Physician Addiction and Impairment—Current Thinking: A Review." *J Addict Dis* 13, no. 1 (1994): 91–105.

22. Brooke, D., G. Edwards, and C. Taylor. "Addiction as an Occupational Hazard: 144 Doctors with Drug and Alcohol Problems." *Brit J Addict* 86, no. 8 (1991): 1011–1016. https://doi.org/10.1111/j.1360-0443.1991.tb01862.x

23. American Medical Association. "AMA Code of Medical Ethics Opinion 9.3.2: Physician Responsibilities to Impaired Colleagues." November 14, 2016. https://www.ama-assn.org/delivering-care/ethics/physician-responsibilities-impaired-colleagues

24. DesRoches, C.M., S.R. Rao, J.A. Fromson, R.J. Birnbaum, L. Iezzoni, C. Vogeli, and E.G. Campbell. "Physicians' Perceptions, Preparedness for Reporting, and Experiences Related to Impaired and Incompetent Colleagues." *JAMA* 304, no. 2 (2010): 187–193. https://doi.org/10.1001/jama.2010.921

25. "The Sick Physician: Impairment by Psychiatric Disorders, including Alcoholism and Drug Dependence." *JAMA* 223, no. 6 (1973): 684–687.

26. Candilis, P.J., D.T. Kim, and L.S. Sulmasy. "Physician Impairment and Rehabilitation: Reintegration Into Medical Practice While Ensuring Patient Safety: A Position Paper From the American College of Physicians." *Ann Intern Med* 170, no. 12 (2019): 871–879. https://doi.org/10.7326/M18-3605

27. Boyd, J.W. "Deciding Whether To Refer a Colleague to a Physician Health Program." *AMA J Ethics* (2015): 888–893.

28. The Council on Science and Public Health. "Report 1 of The Council on Science and Public Health (I-10) Physician Health Programs." *American Medical Association/* 2010. https://www.ama-assn.org/sites/ama-assn.org/files/corp/media-browser/public/about-ama/councils/Council%20Reports/council-on-science-public-health/i10-csaph-model-programs-physician-health.pdf

29. McLellan, A.T., G.E. Skipper, M. Campbell, and R.L. DuPont. "Five Year Outcomes in a Cohort Study of Physicians Treated for Substance Use Disorders in the United States." *BMJ* 337 (2008). https://doi.org/10.1136/bmj.a2038

30. DuPont, R.L., A.T. McLellan, G. Carr, M. Gendel, and G.E. Skipper. "How Are Addicted Physicians Treated? A National Survey of Physician Health Programs." *J Subst Abuse Treat* 37, no. 1 (2009): 1–7. https://doi.org/10.1016/j.jsat.2009.03.010

13
Spirituality, Religion, and Humanism

Medical professionals began to discuss the responsibility to work proactively toward patient-centered care and quality improvement long ago (see Chapter 6 of this volume). Current medical guidelines include making care more accessible, reliable, and collaborative. Medical professionals delivering patient-centered care are called to be compassionate and constructive members of the healthcare system. Not only that, but medical ethics requires respect for the religious and spiritual beliefs of others and for the medical professional to be cognizant of the dynamics involved when interacting with patients. However, medical professionals also have a right to their own personal beliefs, while maintaining a primary obligation to their patients.

This chapter has three goals:

1. To provide an abbreviated review of the role of religion, spirituality, and humanism in medicine.
2. To discuss medical professionals' approaches to spiritual subjects in a patient-centered practice.
3. To emphasize the importance of health professionals attending to their own spiritual beliefs, even in the professional setting.

The history of religion in medicine

Although it may be hard to imagine in this age of evidence-based, competency-driven healthcare, medicine and religion were integrated for thousands of years. Ancient civilizations throughout the Afro-Eurasian supercontinent believed sickness had supernatural causes. Religious rituals were common healing practices for many types of ailments, and hospitals did not exist in Western civilization until the end of the classical period.

The first hospitals were built at the insistence of religious leaders. St. Basil, bishop of Caesarea, had a hospital built in Asia Minor in 370 CE, and Hsiao Tzu-Liang, a Buddhist prince, founded the first hospital in China in 491 CE. Monks and priests were the primary healers throughout the Middle Ages, and the Church was crucial in the provision of medical care. Progressively, over the next few centuries, through the Renaissance and Enlightenment periods, Western medicine shifted toward primarily scientifically based practices.[1]

Current trends of religion in healthcare

Religion still plays a crucial role in American medicine today. Many hospitals and healthcare systems still have religious affiliations or at least bear the religious monikers that they have carried for decades. Examples include the Houston Methodist Hospital, Barnes-Jewish Hospital, and the Ascension healthcare system. Catholic hospitals currently represent 10 of the 25 major hospital systems in the United States. Furthermore, while the number of public hospitals and other nonprofit health systems has declined, the number of Catholic hospitals rose by 16 percent between 2001 and 2011.[2]

Providing compassionate care for the sick and wounded is a central tenet of many religious ideologies, and religious hospitals and doctors look to their faith for motivation and inspiration. Additionally, despite a growing trend toward secularization in many areas of American life, patients are still more likely to be religious than not. According to a survey by the Pew Research Center, 65 percent of Americans surveyed defined themselves as Christian, 7 percent practiced non-Christian faiths, and those who describe their religious affiliation as "Nothing in Particular" represented 26 percent of the U.S. population surveyed. [3] And because religion is a personal experience, each person carries their beliefs with a varied amount of fervor and commitment. Nevertheless, one's beliefs will likely, in some way, affect healthcare priorities and choices, as well as the way they cope with diagnoses and complications.

Spirituality

Being *religious* is not necessary for a patient to have beliefs that influence care. The patient may instead describe their personal beliefs as spiritual. Although spirituality and religion are often used interchangeably in medical

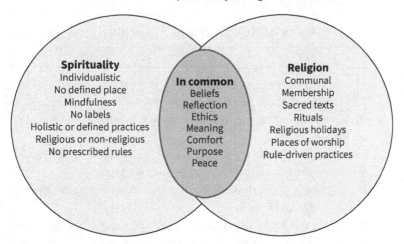

Figure 13.1 The intersection between spirituality and religion.

literature, they are not necessarily the same. There are many definitions and ways of drawing contrast between these two terms, but for our purposes, religion is an organized system of beliefs, practices and symbols that connect humans to a higher power, while spirituality is "the aspect of humanity that refers to the way individuals seek and express meaning and purpose and the way they experience their connectedness to the moment, to self, to others, to nature, and to the significant or sacred."[4p887] One does not have to be religious to be spiritual, and vice versa. It is helpful to keep this in mind when learning about a patient's beliefs or faith, as you may find yourself asking the wrong questions if you believe that only those who are religious are spiritual or that some set amount of spirituality comes with being religious. We all find meaning in different ways, and it is necessary to keep an open mind and realize that there may be ways of being spiritual or religious with which we are not familiar or may not have previously encountered. Figure 13.1 highlights the overlap between spirituality and religion.

The impact of faith and spirituality on health

Before a religious patient even steps into the clinic, their faith has an impact on their health. The effects of religion on a person's subjective well-being are generally widespread and positive (Box 13.1).[5]

Box 13.1 **Effects of Religion and Spirituality on Health**

- Believing in a higher power or a guiding set of principles in the universe helps produce a calming effect and reduce stress.
- Social support from churches, synagogues, temples, mosques, or other religious community centers improves health outcomes and reduces mortality.
- Prayer and meditation induce the relaxation response, which can improve many health indicators through mental tranquility.
- The practice of religion will have an impact on your patients through faith, worship, and prayer.
- Religion is often seen as a protective factor with an inverse predictive relationship to suicide and mortality along with anxiety and depression.[6]

Once inside the clinic, religious faith is often felt less acutely because many physicians do not feel comfortable discussing their own or patients' religious beliefs, or they choose not to address them for other reasons. However, patients want their physicians to consider their religious and spiritual beliefs. One study revealed that the number of respondents who wanted physicians to ask about spiritual beliefs was 83 percent, citing a desire for understanding between the physician and patient. Patients stated a belief that the understanding of their spiritual beliefs would encourage realistic hope by the physician (67 percent), affect the physician's ability to give medical advice (66 percent), and change treatment (62 percent).[7]

It is clear that many patients want their faith to be considered by physicians in all settings. Do physicians feel adequately prepared to engage in this discussion? They may not know how to broach the topic, or they may feel that they are not familiar enough with a patient's religion to discuss it without risking umbrage. However, like cultural praxis, physicians must be willing to humbly admit ignorance and learn to ask appropriate, respectful questions that do not project bias. Physicians may also avoid talking about faith because they feel pressured by time restrictions they see as limiting their ability to discuss anything not directly related to patient care. But many patients want to discuss their beliefs with their physicians, and a failure to do so may negatively impact the patient's experience and outcomes. A few ways for physicians to effectively engage in interventions that target specific spiritual beliefs of patients in accordance with the health belief model are provided in Table 13.1.

Although a patient's faith is usually associated with an increase in the ability to cope, it can sometimes become maladaptive and contribute to feelings of anxiety, hopelessness, and depression that may occur after receiving bad news from a clinician. The struggle between a patient's meaning of life and the variation in meaning that a diagnosis or procedure can pose may also induce posttraumatic stress symptoms.[8] Depending on the patient and circumstances, some may view illness as a punishment from God.[9] It can be extremely challenging for a patient to go through the disease process while also feeling estranged from a belief system. Serious diagnoses, prognoses, or outcomes may lead to a sense of hopelessness regarding religion and God, which can further plague a patient's attempt to come to terms with the situation.

Studies have shown that patients with life-changing diagnoses (primarily cancer) have a higher quality of life if they remain optimistic.[10] On the other hand, patients who feel that they can no longer stand by their religion may lose their optimistic belief in an overarching plan or a benevolent God, and this in turn can result in a lower quality of life.[11] These outcomes are unfortunate in and of themselves, and they can also lead to increased morbidity and mortality during the recovery period after surgical operations. Therefore, helping patients cope with the difficulties involved in medical procedures is within your purview as a physician, even if this necessitates religious discussion.[12] A physician who can competently attend to the spiritual needs of patients may produce better health outcomes than one who attempts to treat only the body and neglects the mind and soul.

You may be wondering whether nonreligious spirituality has the same benefits as religion on health outcomes. There is some evidence that certain spiritual practices can provide the benefits of religion. Those who are highly spiritual and invested in finding meaning and purpose in life may have similar coping strategies, and therefore benefits, to patients who look to their religion for comfort when they are experiencing trauma. For example, nonreligious spiritual patients who choose to meditate to connect with their sense of meaning can trigger the *relaxation response,* which can have positive effects on many health indicators.[13] Meditation, whether practiced

Table 13.1 Targeting Spiritual Beliefs in Primary Care

Health Belief Model Factor	Spiritual Belief(s)	Interventions
Perceived severity: How serious is this illness?	• I'll pray that it gets better • Use of spiritual remedies (e.g. salves, fasting) may delay seeking medical attention	Providers may engage patients in dialogue about their beliefs while providing information about treatment and alternatives.
4Perceived susceptibility: What is the risk of contracting illness?	• God is in control. • Fatalism/everything happens for a reason	Providers may provide information about health risk in community and faith-based organizations as well as to individual patients.
Perceived benefits: Is treatment feasible? Efficacious?	• My body is a temple • I want to live longer • God helps those who help themselves • My church values health	Use of faith-based promotional materials. Referrals to chaplains/faith-based organizations to promote healthy practices.
Perceived barriers: Cost-benefit, practical concerns.	• My beliefs prevent me from engaging in certain health behaviors or practices (i.e. contraception, organ donation)	Engage in dialogue and allow patients to express concerns. If needed, make referrals to chaplains/faith-based organizations to help patient arrive at decisions that take their beliefs into consideration.
Self –efficacy: Ability to execute desired behavior	• Higher power (i.e. God) gives me the power/courage to do anything • God is in control • Do my spiritual beliefs support what I want to do?	Partnerships between clinics and community/faith organizations may promote healthy behaviors and engagement with primary-care facilities.
Cues to action: Triggers to taking action	• Announcements about other church members who have fallen ill • Preexisting health conditions	Providers may provide workshops in the community/churches to increase health awareness.
Socio-psychological variables	• Social support in church	

Reprinted by permission from Springer Nature: *Journal of Religion and Health* 55, no. 3 (June 2016): 1065–1077, "Incorporating Spirituality in Primary Care," by K.S. Isaac, J.L. Hay, and E.I. Lubetkin, © 2016.

spiritually (focusing on a word such as "om," "peace," or "love") or religiously (choosing instead "Insha'Allah," "Sh'ma Yisroel," or "The Lord is my shepherd"), can lead to decreased metabolism, heart rate, blood pressure, and muscle tension through the relaxation response.[14] It may be effective in the treatment of many conditions, such as hypertension, chronic pain, anxiety, and insomnia.

Tools to obtain patients' views on faith and spirituality

Discussing religion and spirituality with patients ought to be approached with care to ensure that professional boundaries are not overstepped. For physicians who feel uncomfortable discussing religion or spirituality in a free-form manner with their patients, there are tools for obtaining information in a systematic way that can be administered by members of the clinical team. Once the information is obtained, a decision can be made on how to garner further information to integrate into care. The two tools we describe in this chapter are the HOPE Questions for Spiritual Assessment and the FICA Spiritual Assessment Tool.

The HOPE questions cover religion, spirituality, and individual sources of meaning that may not be considered religious or spiritual.[15] HOPE is an acronym that helps physicians easily remember how to navigate discussions of faith and beliefs. The letters stand for

H: Sources of hope, meaning, comfort, strength, peace, love, and connection.
O: Organized religion.
P: Personal spirituality and practices.
E: Effects on medical care and end-of-life issues.

The HOPE questions are flexible and simply serve as a guideline. Depending on patients' answers, physicians may modify the questions asked in subsequent sections. For example, if a patient mentions that their involvement in their Baptist church is the major source of hope and meaning in her life, many of the "O" questions can be skipped, with the "P" questions used to tease out the patient's specific beliefs or relationship with God. If a patient details their spiritual practices when describing their sources of strength and peace, then the "P" questions can be foregone, and the "O" questions may be more important for determining if these practices follow any organized religious teachings or if they are more personal, self-directed beliefs. In this way, the HOPE questions can help physicians move quickly through the pertinent aspects of a patient's beliefs and perspectives and even how they might affect treatment. Using the "E" questions effectively, physicians can get direct, candid answers to how faith could impact methods and outcomes.

The FICA Spiritual Assessment Tool is a similar method for analyzing a patient's beliefs and how they might apply to their medical care.[16] Although it is called a "spiritual" assessment tool, it may be used to obtain both spiritual and religious information. Like HOPE, FICA is an acronym designed to help doctors easily remember the necessary components of inquiry. FICA stands for

F: Faith and belief.
I: Importance.
C: Community.
A: Address in care.

The FICA Spiritual Assessment Tool differs from the HOPE questions in a few ways. The "F" in of FICA is a combination of the "H" and "O" questions of HOPE, while the "I" and "C" aspects of FICA seek to glean information about what aspects of spirituality and religion are most important to the patient. Despite these differences, both are effective methods for guiding the conversation about religion and spirituality and take about 10 to 20 minutes to administer. It is probably best to try both and determine which one works for you in your practice and to personalize the questions so that they are more individualized for you and your patients.

Helping patients discuss their views on religion and spirituality to improve the patient experience and improve outcomes may be easier than you think. As a physician, you already discuss the most personal physical and mental aspects of a patient's life and do so professionally and without judgment. With a bit more effort, clinicians can learn to use this practiced bedside manner in a way that will make patients feel comfortable discussing religion and spirituality. However, keep in mind that some patients may not want to discuss their faith during a visit to the clinic.

Although many patients are interested in sharing their faith with their physicians, others believe that the hospital or doctor's office is not an appropriate setting for such a discussion, and that is fine. Do not attempt to coerce reticent patients into discussing their beliefs. Physicians ought to keep in mind the tenets of active listening: making eye contact, giving affirmations, and asking questions when appropriate, as well as being careful not to interrupt the speaker (see Chapter 6 of this volume). By combining active listening and a nonjudgmental demeanor, physicians can make it easier for patients to discuss their beliefs. It is important for physicians to respond in a nonjudgmental, respectful way, because even patients who wish to discuss their faith may experience vulnerability by choosing to open up. By practicing patient-centered communication, the physician–patient relationship may be strengthened rather than eroded.

Crucially, physicians should also be familiar with resources for referring patients to religious leaders or experts who may be able to help them further with any questions they have about how their treatment relates to their beliefs or religious teachings. Just as a heart specialist can perform cardiac procedures more precisely than a general practitioner, an experienced priest, rabbi, chaplain, or other religious leaders will be able to answer questions of theology more accurately than we can. For some patients, these resources may be beneficial for their peace of mind during the disease process.

Physicians' personal faith and beliefs

We have highlighted tools to help physicians navigate patient consultations concerning religion and spiritually. But how does a physician's faith affect the way they practice medicine? Can physicians continue to practice their faith and live by their beliefs while continuing to follow ethical and professional principles?

Physicians are, of course, all different. While they must all be knowledgeable, professional, and committed to health outcomes, there is a tremendous amount of wiggle room within these requirements. Some physicians are more collaborative, while others are more prescriptive. And they all have different styles. Likewise, many physicians possess unique religious and spiritual beliefs. A study conducted by the University of Chicago showed that 70 percent of physicians are religious.[17]

Physician beliefs may affect healthcare by influencing which procedures they are willing to carry out, recommend, or condone.[18] Physicians' religious ideologies might also affect how they interact with patients or what they prioritize in their practice, depending on whether their faith emphasizes charity, family, or any number of other qualities. Religion plays a significant role in the lives of many patients and physicians, and it may be inextricable from the patient–physician interaction. As a physician, it will be important to learn how to manage, balance, and utilize both your and your patients' faiths.

It is possible to be true to your faith while working within the healthcare environment of the United States, as long as the well-being of the patient remains the main priority. According to the AMA, it *may* be ethically permissible for physicians to decline a potential patient when specific treatments sought are incompatible with the physician's deeply held personal, religious, or moral beliefs.[19] Yet, every state and institution has established their own code of ethics, which may differ from the AMA's opinion. In some cases, your role as a professional may require you to act against your personal beliefs, such as in an emergency when someone needs life-saving care rendered immediately. The priority should always be patient safety, but as long as your personal beliefs do not interfere with that goal, there should not be issues with abiding by your own religion or spirituality in the clinical environment.

Humanism in medicine

Humanism has taken root in medicine as a foundation for respectful and compassionate relationships between physicians and their patients. Humanism is a philosophical stance that emphasizes the value and agency of humans. This philosophy has existed and been transformed over the centuries. Major development occurred during the Renaissance and Enlightenment periods as scholars conceptualized that human virtue could result from human reason alone, independent from God or gods or any religious institutions.[20] In the mid-20th century, humanistic psychology rose to prominence as a counterpoint to the psychoanalytic theory of Sigmund Freud and the behavioral theory of B. F. Skinner. Humanistic psychology highlights the natural desire for self-actualization said to be present in all humans, drawing from the humanistic theories of the Renaissance and Enlightenment. As a response to the dehumanizing pressures of technology in medicine, the ideals of humanism in medicine were developed by pediatric neurologist Arnold Gold in 1988 with Sandra Gold and other colleagues at Columbia University's College of Physicians and Surgeons.[21] Many different concepts that are in use today are derived from the Latin root of *humanitas* (see Table 13.2).

Table 13.2 Current Beliefs That Are Shaped by Humanism

Category	Core Beliefs	Examples
Humanism in medicine	• Integrity, excellence, collaboration & compassion, altruism, respect and resilience, empathy, service (I.E., C.A.R.E.S.) • Respectful and empathic physician–patient relationship • Care that reflects an understanding of the attitudes, behaviors, and backgrounds of patients	Has roots in the Hippocratic Oath and from the 1500s; currently being taught in medical schools and moved forward by the Gold Foundation (https://www.gold-foundation.org/)
Humanistic psychology	• A reaction to psychoanalytic and behavioral theories that posits that humans are inherently good and have a drive toward self-actualization • Encourages self-awareness and mindfulness in order to allow the patient to change their thoughts and behaviors • Acknowledges the importance of spiritual aspiration as part of the psyche	Carl Rogers, Otto Rank, and Abraham Maslow were some of the progenitors of this theory.
Medical humanities	• Fosters humanistic principles by studying literature, art, philosophy, ethics, film, and other related disciplines • Develops humanism in healthcare practitioners	Many UME and GME programs incorporate medical humanities into the curriculum.
Secular humanism	• Focuses on humanistic values without the framework of an organized religion • Posits that humans have an intrinsic capability for morality and reason without existence of a God or gods	The founder of the Council for Secular Humanim, Paul Kurtz
Religious humanism	• Incorporates humanistic values into a religious institution	As many as half or more Unitarian Universalists identify as humanists (https://www.uua.org/)
Christian humanism	• Incorporates the beliefs of universal human dignity and that individuals have the capacity for self-improvement into the framework of Christianity • Advocates study of classical ideas and texts	Much of the foundational thought draws from the works of Erasmus from the northern Renaissance

In developing the idea of medical humanism, Sandra Gold and her colleagues feared that new scientific discoveries and technology were transforming medicine to be overly reliant on technology rather than focused on the whole patient. The Gold Foundation states that humanism in healthcare "reflects attitudes and behaviors that are sensitive to the values and the cultural and ethnic backgrounds of others."[21] The humanistic physician demonstrates the attributes of "I.E. C.A.R.E.S":

- *Integrity*: The congruence between expressed values and behavior.
- *Excellence*: Clinical expertise.
- *Collaboration and compassion*: The awareness and acknowledgement of the suffering of another and the desire to relieve it.
- *Altruism*: The capacity to put the needs and interests of another before your own.
- *Respect and resilience*: The regard for the autonomy and values of another person.
- *Empathy*: The ability to put oneself in another's situation (e.g., physician as patient).
- *Service*: The sharing of one's talent, time and resources with those in need; giving beyond what is required.

To foster humanism early in the training of medical professionals, the Gold Foundation created the white-coat ceremony to welcome new medical students and to set clear expectations of their primary role as physicians. This ceremony has been adopted by 99 percent of allopathic medical schools in the United States. In it, matriculating medical students recite the Hippocratic Oath, or a different profession of values, before they even begin their first day of classes, to understand their responsibilities to learn the values of humanism and serve as humanistic physicians. The Gold Foundation also established the Gold Humanism Honor Society, comprising over 25,000 healthcare professionals who have been recognized for practicing patient-centered care.

So why, exactly, has the Gold Foundation focused so much on instilling the values of humanism in our medical professionals? They have identified four concrete improvements in medicine that result from humanistic care, which they call the Quadruple Aim:[22]

- Better experience.
- Better health.
- Lower cost.
- Joy of work.

The research supporting these aims can be found online in the Gold Database of Research.[23]

One study found that Gold Humanism Honor Society members scored significantly higher in measures of clinical empathy, patient-centered beliefs, and tolerance of ambiguity while maintaining higher levels of empathy and patient-centeredness throughout medical school.[24] Because these values are implicated in delivering better patient care, continuing to create curricula that emphasize the development of humanism seems to be a reasonable goal for medical training programs. A movement toward humanism in medicine may also be part of the solution to the physician burnout epidemic. By ensuring that physicians find more meaning in their work while simultaneously increasing the efficiency of the healthcare delivery process, humanism may improve overall physician happiness and well-being.

Chapter Quick Summary

- Medical professionals have a responsibility to work proactively toward patient-centered care and consistent quality improvement, which includes respecting the religious and spiritual values of patients.
- Religion has been a significant part of medicine for centuries and continues to have a presence within a number of current healthcare institutions.
- Spirituality can be religious or nonreligious, and the commonalities of religion and spirituality make it possible to approach patients in a meaningful way guided by shared attributes.
- Spirituality and religion have positive effects on health, for example, through calming effects from meditation and prayer.

- There are two tools provided for physicians to begin obtaining information about the religious and spiritual beliefs of patients: the HOPE Questions for Spiritual Assessment and the FICA Spiritual Assessment Tool.
- The medical professional must decide what, if any, impact their personal beliefs have on their personal and professional lives.
- Humanism has taken root in medicine as a foundation for respectful and compassionate relationships between physicians and their patients.

Resources

Ackerknecht, E.H., and L. Haushofer. *A Short History of Medicine*. Baltimore, MD: Johns Hopkins University Press, 2016.

Arnold P. Gold Foundation. "Gold Humanism Honor Society." https://www.goldfoundation.org/programs/ghhs/

De Oliveira, J.A.C., M.I.P. Anderson, G. Lucchetti, E.V.A. Pires, and L.M. Gonçalves. "Approaching Spirituality Using the Patient-Centered Clinical Method." *J Relig Health* 58, no. 1 (2019): 109–118.

Ehman, J. "Religious Diversity: Practical Points for Health Care Providers." *Penn Medicine*. May 8, 2012. http://www.uphs.upenn.edu/pastoral/resed/diversity_points.html

Shinall, M.C., Jr. "The Separation of Church and Medicine." *Virtual Mentor* 11, no. 10 (2009): 747–749. https://doi.org/10.1001/virtualmentor.2009.11.10.fred1-0910

University of Washington, Department of Bioethics and Humanities. "Spirituality and Medicine." https://depts.washington.edu/bhdept/ethics-medicine/bioethics-topics/detail/79

References

1. Koenig, H.G. "Religion and Medicine I: Historical Background and Reasons for Separation." *Intl J Psychiatr Med* 30, no. 4 (2000): 385–398.
2. Friedman, L. "Dispelling Six Myths About Catholic Hospital Care in the United States." *Rewire*. June 24, 2014. https://rewire.news/article/2014/06/24/dispelling-six-myths-catholic-hospital-care-united-states/

3. Pew Research Center. "In U.S., Decline of Christianity Continues at Rapid Pace." *Religion & Public Life.* October 17, 2019. https://www.pewforum.org/2019/10/17/in-u-s-decline-of-christianity-continues-at-rapid-pace/

4. Puchalski, C., B. Ferrell, R. Virani, S. Otis-Green, P. Baird, J. Bull, H. Chochinov, G. Handzo, H. Nelson-Becker, M. Prince-Paul, and K. Pugliese. "Improving the Quality of Spiritual Care as a Dimension of Palliative Care: The Report of the Consensus Conference." *J Palliat Med* 12, no. 10 (2009): 885–904.

5. Villani, D., A. Sorgente, P. Iannello, and A. Antonietti. "The Role of Spirituality and Religiosity in Subjective Well-Being of Individuals with Different Religious Status." *Front Psychol* 10 (2019), https://doi.org/10.3389/fpsyg.2019.01525

6. Pugh, K. "Religious Attendance, Surrender to God, and Suicide Risk: Mediating Pathways of Feeling Forgiven by God and Psychopathology." *Electronic Theses and Dissertations* 3535 (2019). https://dc.etsu.edu/etd/3535

7. McCord, G., V.J. Gilchrist, S.D. Grossman, B.D. King, K.F. McCormick, A.M. Oprandi, S.L. Schrop, B.A. Selius, W.D. Smucker, D.L. Weldy, and M. Amorn. "Discussing Spirituality with Patients: A Rational and Ethical Approach." *Ann Fam Med* 2, no. 4 (2004): 356–361.

8. Appel, J.E., C.L. Park, J.H. Wortmann, and H.T. van Schie. "Meaning Violations, Religious/spiritual Struggles, and Meaning in Life in the Face of Stressful Life Events." *Intl J Psychol Relig* 30, no. 1 (2020): 1–17.

9. Grill, K.B., J. Wang, Y.I. Cheng, and M.E. Lyon. "The Role of Religiousness and Spirituality in Health-related Quality of Life of Persons Living with HIV: A Latent Class Analysis." *Psychol Relig Spirit* 12 (2020). https://doi.org/10.1037/rel0000301

10. Arora, K. *Spirituality and Meaning Making in Chronic Illness: How Spiritual Caregivers Can Help People Navigate Long-term Health Conditions.* London: Jessica Kingsley, 2020.

11. Deimling, G.T., K.F. Bowman, S. Sterns, L.J. Wagner, and B. Kahana. "Cancer-related Health Worries and Psychological Distress among Older Adult, Long-term Cancer Survivors." *Psycho-Oncology* 15, no. 4 (2016): 306–320.

12. Tully, P.J., and R.A. Baker. "Depression, Anxiety, and Cardiac Morbidity Outcomes after Coronary Artery Bypass Surgery: A Contemporary and Practical Review." *J Geriat Cardiol* 9, no. 2 (2012): 197.

13. Benson, H., and M.Z. Klipper. *The Relaxation Response.* New York: Morrow, 1975.

14. Galvin, J.A., H. Benson, G.R. Deckro, G.L. Fricchione, and J.A. Dusek. "The Relaxation Response: Reducing Stress and Improving Cognition in Healthy Aging Adults." *Complement Ther Clin Pract* 12, no. 3 (2016): 186–191. https://doi.org/10.1016/j.ctcp.2006.02.004

15. Anandarajah, G., and E. Hight, "Spirituality and Medical Practice: Using the HOPE Questions as a Practical Tool for Spiritual Assessment." *Amer Fam Physician* 63, no. 1, (2001): 81–89.

16. McSherry, W., L. Ross, K. Balthip, N. Ross, and S. Young. "Spiritual Assessment in Healthcare: An Overview of Comprehensive, Sensitive Approaches to Spiritual Assessment for Use within the Interdisciplinary Healthcare Team." In *Spirituality in Healthcare: Perspectives for Innovative Practice*. Edited by F. Timmins and S. Caldeira, 39–54. Cham, Switzerland: Springer, 2019.

17. Curlin, F.A., J.D. Lantos, C.J. Roach, S.A. Sellergren, and M.H. Chin. "Religious Characteristics of U.S. Physicians: A National Survey." *J Gen Inter Med* 20, no. 7 (2005): 629–634. https://doi.org/10.1111/j.1525-1497.2005.0119.x

18. Curlin, F.A., M.H. Chin, S.A. Sellergren, C.J. Roach, and J.D. Lantos. "The Association of Physicians' Religious Characteristics with Their Attitudes and Self-Reported Behaviors Regarding Religion and Spirituality in the Clinical Encounter." *Med Care* 44, no. 5 (2006): 446–453.

19. American Medical Association. "Code of Medical Ethics Opinion 1.1.2 Prospective Patients." November 14, 2016. https://www.ama-assn.org/delivering-care/ethics/prospective-patients

20. Grendler, P. "Humanism." *Oxford Bibliographies Online*. Last updated June 27, 2017. https://doi.org/10.1093/obo/9780195399301-0002

21. Gold Foundation. "About Us: FAQs." https://www.gold-foundation.org/about-us/faqs/

22. Arnold P. Gold Foundation. "Humanism in Healthcare Supports the Quadruple Aim." https://www.gold-foundation.org/programs/research/quadruple-aim/

23. Arnold P. Gold Foundation. "Gold Database of Research." https://www.gold-foundation.org/resources/databases/gold-database-of-research/.

24. Gaufberg, E., L. Dunham, E. Krupat, B. Stansfield, C. Christianson, and S. Skochelak. "Do Gold Humanism Honor Society Inductees Differ From Their Peers in Empathy, Patient-Centeredness, Tolerance of Ambiguity, Coping Style, and Perception of the Learning Environment?" *Teach Learn Med* 30, no. 3 (2018): 284–293. https://doi.org/10.1080/10401334.2017.1419873

14

Personal Financial Considerations for Physicians

Physicians in the United States are compensated well, with an average salary of $208,000 in 2019 according to the Bureau of Labor Statistics.[1] However, most physicians begin practice with significant financial burdens. The traditional path to becoming a physician involves completing a four-year undergraduate degree, a four-year medical school program, three to seven years of residency, and, potentially, one to three years of a fellowship. According to the American Association of Medical Colleges (AAMC), the median debt of indebted medical student graduates was $200,000 in 2019. Of those who graduated medical school, 73 percent were in debt, and 54 percent of those with debt owed over $200,000, while 18 percent owed over $300,000.[2] Furthermore, when you take into account the potential lost wages from years spent in medical school and residency, it is evident that entering the field of medicine is perhaps not as lucrative as it may seem at first.

Without a solid financial plan, the burden of debt can add significant stress to an already demanding career. Regardless of where you are along in your career, there are considerations to take about your finances. While money is not the only key to happiness (see Chapter 3 of this volume), mismanaging it can certainly lead to anxiety and decreased quality of life. Debt and lack of financial preparedness have been shown to be associated with stress and burnout in trainees. Poor financial planning may also lead to decreased patient outcomes by forcing aging physicians to continue working. It is therefore part of our responsibility as medical professionals to manage our finances and learn the best practices for financial literacy. Furthermore, the paradigms of physician reimbursement continue to change in the United States as healthcare continues to experience disruptive forces. This chapter will provide a brief overview of the personal financial considerations associated with being a physician and resources for maintaining financial health.

Current issues regarding physicians' personal finances

In general, physicians work hard to become experts in everything they undertake, but many do not develop an expertise level of financial literacy. A lack of education on how to manage debt and save money in medical school and residencies inadequately prepares young physicians who require these skills throughout the rest of their lives. Many students choose to specialize in more lucrative specialties due to the perceived pressure of educational debt, contributing to a shortage of primary care physicians. Many physicians adopt poor financial habits as soon as they receive their first paycheck after residency. They may not understand the various retirement plans that are available to them or about the time-value of money in investing. Regardless of the causes, poor financial literacy persists in the medical profession. This is worrying, not only for the financial health of physicians, but also for the well-being of their patients.

Poor financial planning leads to later retirement and a lower standard of care

Because of poor financial planning, many physicians are retiring later than they would like. Not only can this be detrimental to the well-being of the physician, but it can also be detrimental to their patients' health (see Chapter 15 of this volume). There are serious ethical considerations at play. One study examined the link between physician age and patient mortality rates and found that patients treated by older physicians have significantly higher 30-day mortality rates.[3] In fact, their findings suggest that within the same hospital, patients treated by physicians under the age of 40 have an 11 percent lower probability of dying compared with patients cared for by physicians aged 60 and over. The authors of the study speculate that this is because of effects due to aging and training differences.

A major dilemma arises when an older physician cannot maintain the standard of care expected of all physicians, yet is not able to retire because of financial reasons. For physicians to prepare for the future financially, it is important to begin planning for retirement while they are still young. Each additional year of compounding interest is valuable for retirement. Because most physicians begin their careers with substantial debt and little to no savings, saving for retirement is often put on the back burner to address the more pressing issue of paying off loans. However, this is not a wise strategy. Creating a debt management plan that combines repayment and retirement savings is crucial for long-term financial security.

Medical students and residents are, in general, not financially literate

We train our physicians to be brilliant thinkers, scientists, and clinicians and assume that the critical thinking skills we instill in them in medical school and residency will extend to all their endeavors, including financial matters. However, this is not the case. According to the 2017 Report on U.S. Physicians' Financial Preparedness, 71 percent of residents admitted that they did not have the skills to plan to pay off their medical debt.[4]

Young doctors often do not start thinking about their finances until they are attending physicians, when significant student loan interest may have already accrued. Neither residents nor medical school students feel financially prepared, although even the most basic training could help significantly. In a study of senior medical school students, the majority felt that a 3.5 hour workshop on financial literacy was useful, and 64 percent of students felt that the session provided tools that would be useful in the future.[5] A study that polled 60 radiation oncology residents and 15 program directors at the Jefferson Medical College of Thomas Jefferson University found that 75 percent of residents felt unprepared to handle future financial decisions.[6] Likewise, 80 percent of the directors felt that the residents were unprepared to deal with future financial decisions, but nearly 90 percent of the directors reported that they would be able to adjust program curricula to include lectures on financial topics. It is evident that introducing a financial literacy curriculum for residents and medical students, or even premedical students, would be a viable and effective solution.

Expected future income and current debt influence physicians' decisions to specialize

There is a large disparity in compensation between medical specialties. According to the Merritt Hawkins Incentive Review of 2020, the average starting salary of invasive cardiologists was $640,000, while average starting salary for family medicine was $240,000.[7] This disparity in compensation influences young physicians' decisions to specialize. In a study involving medical students at New York Medical College and East Carolina University's Brody School of Medicine, surveys asking questions about career choice, income, and debt were administered to first-year students scheduled to graduate between 1996 and 2012 and fourth-year students graduating between 1993 and 2010.[8] This study found that students intending to go into nonprimary care specialties as compared to students intending to go into primary care anticipated, on average, greater debt of $29,237 (year 1) or $24,904 (year 4), placed a higher importance on income, and anticipated earning an average of $58,463 (year 1) and $89,909 (year 4) more after graduation.

Another study at the University of Toronto Medical School found that students from each year were able to accurately predict income by specialty and that 85 to 89 percent of students in each class feel that family physicians were not paid enough.[9] A study of medical school graduates reported an inverse relationship between debt and intention to enter primary care, especially for students who owed more than $150,000.[10] This is a trend that is supported by current data; the AAMC expects the shortage of primary care physicians to grow to between 7,300 and 43,100 physicians by the year 2030, in which they expect the demand to be for 274,700 physicians.[11] Alarmingly, these numbers already account for the increasing number of nurse practitioners and physician assistants who are beginning to fill the role of the primary care provider (see Chapter 8 of this volume).

Primary care doctors can still pay off debt and save for retirement while living a comfortable life. The key is financial literacy. It is unfortunate that medical students are forgoing their passions to specialize in more lucrative fields. This is certainly not good for the profession and is detrimental to physician well-being and happiness. With more focus on personal finance in medical education, we may be able to reverse the trend of shortages in primary care. Every student has different circumstances that they will have to handle, but by managing their debt and the expectations that they have for their future income and retirement, they will be able to form an accurate vision for their future that can allow them to be financially satisfied, regardless of the specialty they choose.

The gender pay gap and special financial considerations for female physicians

Unfortunately, medicine still has a significant pay gap between men and women. A study found that male physicians earned 13 percent more than female physicians at the outset of the careers.[12] This gap was found to increase over the next eight years to 28 percent, where it stabilized. This data may be influenced by the fact that there are not as many female physicians in some of the higher-paying specialties, but that, in itself, is a problem. It may also be influenced by the fact that more female physicians work part-time (23 percent) than male physicians (4 percent).[13] With the medical student population becoming more female, with over half of entering medical school classes being women, the pay gap should decrease over time, but it is important to be aware of the discrepancy that exists today. However, if the more lucrative specialties continue to be male-dominated and if more females continue to choose to work part-time than their male counterparts, the pay gap may continue to persist.

Managing educational debt

Managing educational debt is a significant concern for many physicians. Ideally, physicians should learn the various options available to them before taking out a loan. Table 14.1 compares several loans that medical students can receive from the federal government. In addition, there are also a variety of private lenders available. Typically, the rates offered by private lenders are higher than those offered by the federal government, but there are also competitive, market-based loans available.

Although it may be difficult to afford monthly payments on debt in residency, an income-driven repayment plan can help. These plans subsidize your payments to match your income.[14] For example, a good option for young physicians is Revised Pay As You Earn (REPAYE), in which the federal government subsidizes 50 percent of all interest above the set monthly payment throughout the repayment period. The monthly payment is generally 10 percent of your monthly discretionary income (the difference between your annual income and 150 percent of the poverty line for your family size). For a resident earning $55,000, the monthly payment would be around $300, and with a $300,000 debt and a typical 6 percent interest rate, the monthly interest would be $1,500.

Table 14.1 Examples of Common Student Loans in 2017

Type of Loan	Interest Rate (%)	Start Payments	Start of Interest Accrual	Other Fees (%)	Who Can Receive This Loan	Limit	Other Information
Direct Stafford Loan (Unsubsidized Stafford Loan)	6	6 months after graduation	Medical school	1.1	Must meet the general eligibility requirements for federal student aid.	$40,500 annually	Rate is variable based on 10-year Treasury note rate.
Direct PLUS Loan	7	6 months after graduation	Medical school	4.3	Must meet the general eligibility requirements for federal student aid.	Limited to cost of attendance minus any other financial aid received.	Rate is variable based on the 10-year Treasury note rate.
Perkins Loan	5	9 months after graduation	9 months after graduation	None	Students with exceptional financial need.	Up to $8,000 per year; total you can borrow as a student is $60,000.	Participating institutions receive funding from government and decide which students have the greatest need.
HRSA Primary Care Loan	5	12 months after graduation	12 months after graduation	None	Students who agree to train and practice in primary care, with a 10-year repayment period; must demonstrate financial need.	Participating institutions allocate funds based on financial need up to cost of attendance.	Students who don't practice in primary care have their loans reverted to a 7% interest rate.

Sources: Bureau of Health Workforce, Health Resources & Services Administration. "School-Based Scholarships and Loans." https://bhw.hrsa.gov/loansscholarships/schoolbasedloans; Federal Student Aid, U.S. Department of Education. "Interest Rates and Fees." https://studentaid.ed.gov/sa/types/loans/interest-rates

In this case, the government would subsidize $600 each month. With REPAYE, the repayment period is 25 years, and any outstanding balance on your federal student loans is forgiven at the end of the repayment period.[15]

Loan forgiveness programs are also an option for some physicians, especially those who are working in the public sector with incomes lower than debt. Public Service Loan Forgiveness offers student loan forgiveness for physicians working under public service employers after 10 years of service. This includes physicians working in not-for-profit public hospitals and other organizations such as academia, the public health sector, and military institutions at the federal, state, local, or tribal level. Consider the case study in Box 14.1.

Box 14.1 Case Study 1

An attending family medicine physician is making $200,000 annually. She has $200,000 in student loan debt with an annual interest rate of 6 percent. She is married, but her spouse does not have an income. The couple has a 30-year mortgage that has a $1,500 monthly payment. They are not pursuing any loan forgiveness options. If they want to pay off their loans as soon as possible but also need to save for retirement, what are their options?

An aggressive approach to saving for retirement could include saving 20 percent of their income, which would be $40,000 annually. They can make a pretax contribution of $18,000 to their 401(k), so their effective tax rate would be 17.6 percent for federal income taxes. With approximately $10,500 in FICA taxes, their net income after taxes and retirement savings would be $117,454, or $9,788 per month.

She could attempt to refinance her student loan so that it has a shorter term and a lower interest rate. Even if she wasn't able to refinance the loan, they could still attempt to pay it off in 5 or 10 years. This would make their budget tighter, but they would pay off their debt sooner and save money. With an interest rate of 6 percent, they would need to pay $3,866.56 monthly to pay off their loan in 5 years or $2,220.41 monthly to pay off their loan in 10 years. Paying $3,866.56 monthly would mean that their annual net income would be $71,055.28 which is a lot lower than their gross income of $200,000, but it is still very possible for a married couple to live on this amount. Paying off their loan in 5 years instead of 10 years would ultimately save them $34,455.58. Placing 20 percent of their income in retirement savings and paying off student loans in five years is an aggressive approach that requires careful financial planning, but it can also lead to financial security in the future.

Financial professionals are less likely to advise young physicians

It is often difficult for young physicians to receive professional financial guidance because they have a negative net worth. The lack of financial guidance is worrying, because early on in their careers is when physicians most need it.

Seventy-one percent of residents in 2017 have medical school debt, and 50 percent of residents have over $200,000 of debt.[4] Sixty-two percent of residents feel that they are "behind" financially for retirement. Residents often don't know what they should do first when juggling paying off their school loans, buying a home, saving for their children's college fund, and saving for retirement. It is recommended that residents secure disability, life, and umbrella liability insurance and have three to six months of living expenses in an emergency fund.[16] After those funds are secured, residents should strive to save 15 to 20 percent of gross income for long-term wealth building such as retirement, saving for a house, and college savings for young children. When evaluating medical school debt, consider the interest rate before deciding whether to accelerate payments on the debt or save the money. Depending on the interest rate of your loan, paying off school loans doesn't always need to be the top priority.

The time-value of money

Medical education is an investment paid upfront that cannot be recouped until training is finished. Similarly, the value of money is directly tied to time because of the power of interest. What this means for physicians is that the sooner that they are debt-free, the more earning power they have and the greater the amount that they can save for retirement.

Compound interest is an extremely powerful force, but ample time is necessary for its power to be realized. As an example, with an average annual interest rate of 8 percent, if you invest just $250 a month starting at age 25, you will accumulate $878,570 by the time you are 65; start at 35, you will accumulate $375,073; or 45, and you will accumulate $148,236. Ideally, one should begin saving for retirement as soon as possible, but for physicians this may be difficult. Therefore, a financial plan should be carefully constructed to manage debt and begin saving for retirement.

A good way to gauge, on average, how much you can make over time from the market is to look at the S&P 500, which tracks the 500 largest, most stable companies in the New York Stock Exchange. From 1992 to 2016, the S&P 500's average annual return was 10.72 percent. However, retirement plans are usually diversified among stock, bond, cash investments, managed futures, private equity funds, and real estate investment trusts, and the average annual rate of return is usually about 5 to 8 percent. Still, remember that investing $250 a month starting at 25 with an 8 percent interest rate will yield $878,570: money uninvested is money lost.

The changing landscape of medicine and its impact on physician compensation

The models of physician compensation continue to change, and these changes have had serious consequences on our health and quality of life. Currently, in the United States, health insurance can be purchased in the private marketplace or, in certain cases, is provided by the government. Private health insurance can be purchased from various for-profit insurance companies or from various nonprofit insurers. According to the Kaiser Family Foundation, nearly 160 million Americans, approximately 49 percent of the population, receive employer-sponsored health insurance.[17] Of these, less than 30 percent choose conventional healthcare plans, which allow the patient the choice of any provider and reimburse based on a fee-for-service plan.[18]

According to the National Health Interview Survey, in 2018, 19.7 percent of adults aged 18 to 64 and 42.5 percent of children aged zero to 17 were covered by public health insurance.[19] There are six major government healthcare programs in the United States[20]:

1. Veterans Health Administration program.
2. State Children's Health Insurance Program.
3. Department of Defense TRICARE and TRICARE for Life programs.
4. Indian Health Service program.
5. Medicare.
6. Medicaid.[20]

Medicare is a federal health insurance program for aged and disabled individuals and is the largest health insurance provider in the country. Medicaid is an assistance program run by state and local governments under federal guidelines that provides health coverage for economically disadvantaged groups.

Reimbursement is provided using a system in which a variety of third-party payers, such as the federal government, are responsible for compensation rather than the single-payer system found in Canada and Europe. The most common form of reimbursement is fee for service, although prospective payment and prepaid health plans are also used. A shortcoming of the fee-for-service model is that it tends to incentivize the quantity, not quality, of care. For this reason, there have been efforts to shift away from this model.

The United States spends the most money on healthcare of any other country in the world, and its healthcare cost is the highest in the world.[21] Yet, the United States healthcare system consistently underperforms relative to other countries on most dimensions of performance, according to data from the Commonwealth Fund. Among the 11 countries studied, the United States ranked last overall.[22]

According to the U.S. Census Bureau, approximately 8.5 percent of the population lacks health insurance as of 2019.[23] Many uninsured people receive healthcare through public clinics, state and local health programs, and private providers that adjust costs using charity money or from other payers, but the lack of insurance can lead to financial hardship in the long run. Many uninsured often delay treatment until it is too late.[23] Even among the insured population covered under private health insurance, the preponderance of high-deductible health plans thwarts timely, consistent healthcare, impedes early diagnoses, and causes delays in proper treatment.

The PPACA and its implications

The Patient Protection and Affordable Care Act (PPACA), colloquially known as "Obamacare," provided major changes in healthcare. First, it changed the way that physicians are compensated, from fee for service to a value-based "payment modifier that provides for differential payment ... based upon the quality of care furnished compared to cost."[24] The immediate impact of this is that most physicians are compensated less than before when they treat Medicare patients. It also gave out billions of dollars to providers who successfully implemented the government's vision of integrated provider networks. Physicians were already moving toward salaried employment from private practice, but the passage of this law has accelerated the process.

The PPACA has removed out-of-pocket costs for free preventative services and provides full Medicare reimbursement for these services to providers, which increased preventative care utilization among Medicare patients in 2010.[25] Because of the increased Medicare patient utilization and full reimbursement for preventive care, there has been an increase in income of primary care providers. Even though some primary care providers are making more money, that doesn't mean that all physicians are. Some physicians are opting out of Medicare/Medicaid because of the low reimbursement rates and the large amount of paperwork that needs to be completely for those patients.

The PPACA aims to change the way that medical care is delivered by introducing a new model called the accountable care organization (ACO). An ACO is a network of physicians and hospitals that share responsibility for providing care to its patients. Under the PPACA, an ACO would agree to manage all the healthcare needs of a minimum of 5,000 Medicare beneficiaries for at least three years. By integrating care, ACOs are expected to drive down costs by eliminating unnecessary procedures and tests, while increasing the quality of care.

MACRA and new payment models

The Centers for Medicare and Medicaid Services implemented the Medicare Access and CHIP Reauthorization Act (MACRA) to improve overall quality of care by providing financial incentives for providers.[26] The two payment options for providers are the merit-based incentive payment system and advanced alternative payment models. With the merit-based incentive payment system, payment adjustments of ±4 percent are determined by a score that is based on quality of care, improvement activities, advancing care information, and cost. With advanced alternative payment models, participants must meet certain qualifications to receive a payment adjustment of +5 percent. These reimbursement models represent a shift away from fee for service toward value-based healthcare.

Cash-only and concierge practices

Physicians who participate in cash only and concierge practices aim to bypass the fee-for-service payment model. In a cash-only practice, the patient directly pays the physician for their services. In a concierge practice, patients pay an annual fee for the services of the physician, and they usually have increased accessibility to their physician. Furthermore, the physician agrees not to take on more than a certain number of patients so that they can focus on their client base.

Hospital employment versus private practice

Money is a huge factor for many physicians when deciding between a salaried employment in a hospital and the flexible income of private practice. Despite the difference in compensation, the recent trend has been toward hospital employment. Many physicians in private practice are tired of the increasing administrative and regulatory burdens and are choosing to focus more on patient care (see Chapter 16 of this volume). Also, young physicians just entering practice are pushing the trend toward salaried employment. Consistency of working hours and a fixed income are often attractive to young physicians trying to balance their lifestyle.

However, the money associated with private practice can be a great benefit. Because physicians in private practice receive a much higher percentage of the gross income than physicians in large groups, they can make a lot more money. However, with many of the governmental and insurance regulations being passed, such as the PPACA, the gap is getting smaller. There is also a significant amount of risk involved with going into private practice.

Being a part of a private practice also means having to deal with medical malpractice lawsuits. Although medical malpractice rates vary widely by specialty and state, paying for insurance against medical malpractice can be a major out-of-pocket cost. According to the AMA, in 2018, OB/GYNs faced premiums between $49,804 in some areas of California and $214,999 in some areas of New York.[27]

Planning for retirement

Regardless of where you are in your career, one of the most important ways to plan for your future is to start saving for retirement. It is best to start saving at a young age so that there is more time for interest to accrue on your investments; but it can be difficult for physicians to save their money during the years of their education. Some exercises can help you to begin thinking about how much you will need to save for retirement (see Box 14.2).

Box 14.2 Retirement Planning Exercises

1. Calculate how much money you need for retirement. Think about what age you'll start, or did start, saving for retirement; at what age you want to retire; your life expectancy; what percentage of your income you will need to sustain your lifestyle; the rate of return you think you will receive on your investments; and the amount of Social Security you think you will receive.

   Let's say you start saving at 30 years old, wish to retire at 70 years old, have a life expectancy of 100 years old, currently make $300,000, want 75 percent of your income during retirement, expect no Social Security benefits, expect inflation to be 3 percent, and expect an investment return of 8 percent. You would need $11,539,026 to retire.

2. Use a retirement calculator online to find out what percentage of your income you need to save annually to have enough money for retirement. See how your monthly contributions change if you start saving at the beginning of your residency rather than after your residency is over.

   If you start at age 30 with no retirement savings, to retire with $11,539,026, you need to save $3,582.35 a month for 40 years and have an 8 percent return on investment. However, if you were able to save 10 percent of your $55,000 income during your three-year residency, then you would have $16,500 in retirement savings already at the age of 30. To retire with $11,539,026, you need to save $3,481.18 monthly for 40 years and have an 8 percent return on investment. Starting off with $16,500 in your savings allows you to spend an extra $101.17 every month for 40 years, which totals $48,561.60.

Types of retirement plans

Even though physicians might start saving for retirement later in their lives, they can become financially secure with the right retirement plan. There are many different plans available. Some are pretax and some are posttax. Some retirement plans are only available through an employer, and others can be set up by yourself. Each employer may choose which retirement plans to offer to their employees. The contribution limits vary from year to year; the most recent guidelines can be easily found at the Internal Revenue Service website (https://www.irs.gov/retirement-plans/plan-sponsor/types-of-retirement-plans).[28]

Simplified Employee Pension and Savings Incentive Match Plan for Employees Individual Retirement Account (SIMPLE) are both individual retirement accounts and often good options for physicians working in smaller practices. These are typically easy to set up and participants control their own accounts. Both have minimal eligibility requirements. An important difference is that, for the Simplified Employee Pension, participants cannot contribute their own money, while for the Savings Incentive Match Plan for Employees Individual Retirement Account, the participant may contribute on a pretax basis through payroll deductions up to a maximum set by the Internal Revenue Service.

In a profit-sharing plan, the employer shares a portion of the profits from the company and places it into the retirement account of the employee. By adding a 401(k) feature, employees can redirect a portion of their wages into the retirement plan through payroll deductions.

In a defined benefit plan, the pension level at retirement age is first calculated, based on factors such as current earnings, employee age, and tenure of service. Then, the amount of annual contribution necessary to reach that level is calculated. The advantage of a defined benefit plan is that it allows for significantly higher annual contribution than the profit-sharing or 401(k) plans, which may be useful if you are a higher earning physician. However, defined benefit plans are often more complex and costly to establish and maintain for the employer.

In addition to the savings in your retirement plan, Social Security is a program that is essentially a safety net for retirement. Employees pay into the program through Federal Insurance Contributions Act (FICA) taxes that are withheld from most paychecks, and when it is time to retire, receive benefits from the program. The amount of benefits that you receive is based on the age you retire and the amount of money you earned while employed. The maximum monthly benefit in 2018 is $3,698, but this is only if you begin receiving benefits at age 70 or older and earned the maximum income taxed by FICA ($128,400 in 2018) for a 35-year period. Most physicians will reach this figure, so it is realistic to expect the maximum payout as long as Social Security continues to exist as a program.

Financial resources for physicians

Medical educators have begun to recognize the importance of financial literacy for physicians. The AAMC has recently launched a Financial Wellness Program, which provides free courses on common financial topics and a multitude of resources for financial literacy. For example, the MedLoans® Organizer and Calculator is designed to help physicians manage their medical loans. Additionally, some medical schools and residency programs have begun offering financial literacy courses. Although the profession is only beginning to catch up, there are many available resources for physicians to develop the tools to be financially healthy, many of which are listed at the end of the chapter.

Chapter Quick Summary

- Physicians are compensated well, but they often incur significant debt and only begin making significant money after years of training.
- Financial strain in physicians may contribute to decreased well-being and burnout, as well as decreased patient outcomes.
- The evidence suggests that many medical school students are choosing to specialize in more lucrative specialties due to the financial pressure of debt; this is contributing to a shortage of primary care physicians.
- Financial literacy is not being taught in medical schools and residency programs, although there is a perceived need.

- It is important for physicians to understand the time value of money, especially because they begin their careers later than most.
- Developing a financial plan that involves both paying off debt and saving for retirement is usually the best course of action.
- The payment models are changing for physicians so it is more important than ever to develop a financial plan.
- There are many resources available for physicians to develop financial literacy.

Resources

Association of American Medical College. "The AAMC Financial Wellness Program." https://students-residents.aamc.org/financial-aid/article/aamcfinancialwellness/

Blueprint Income. "Life Expectancy Calculator." https://www.blueprintincome.com/tools/life-expectancy-calculator-how-long-will-i-live/

Dahle, J.M. "List of Physician Financial Blogs." *Whitecoat Investor*. July 13, 2018. https://www.whitecoatinvestor.com/list-of-physician-financial-blogs/

Dahle, J.M. "Ten Reasons Doctors Spend Too Much Money" [Blog post]. *White Coat Investor*. July 14, 2020. https://www.whitecoatinvestor.com/ten-reasons-doctors-spend-too-much-money/

Financial Aid Office, School of Medicine and Dentistry, University of Rochester. "Resources for Financial Wellness." https://www.urmc.rochester.edu/education/financial-aid-office/financial-wellness.aspx

IBRInfo. "Summary of Income-driven Repayment Plans." http://ibrinfo.org/

Passive Income M.D. [Home page]. https://passiveincomemd.com/

"Retirement Calculator." *Calculator.net*. https://www.calculator.net/retirement-calculator.html

Stanley, Thomas J., and William D. Danko. *The Millionaire Next Door: The Surprising Secrets of America's Wealthy*. Lanham, MD: Taylor Trade, 2010.

Wall Street Physician. [Home page]. https://www.wallstreetphysician.com/

Wall Street Physician. "What Is A Good Savings Rate For Retirement?" [Blog post]. October 4, 2017. https://www.wallstreetphysician.com/good-savings-rate-retirement/

Wealthy Doc. [Home page]. https://wealthydoc.org/

References

1. U.S. Bureau of Labor Statistics. "Physicians and Surgeons: Occupational Outlook Handbook." September 1, 2020. https://www.bls.gov/ooh/healthcare/physicians-and-surgeons.htm#tab-1

2. Association of American Medical Colleges. "Medical Student Education: Debt, Costs, and Loan Repayment Fact Card 2019." 2019. https://store.aamc.org/medical-student-education-debt-costs-and-loan-repayment-fact-card-2019-pdf.html

3. Tsugawa, Y., J.P. Newhouse, A.M. Zaslavsky, D.M. Blumenthal, and A.B. Jena. "Physician Age and Outcomes in Elderly Patients in Hospital in the US: Observational Study." *BMJ* 357 (May 16, 2017): j1797. https://doi.org/10.1136/bmj.j1797

4. AMA Insurance. "2017 Report on Resident Physicians' Financial Preparedness." 2017. https://www.ama-assn.org/residents-students/resident-student-finance/financial-planning-residency-3-take-home-points

5. Liebzeit, J., M. Behler, S. Heron, and S. Santen. "Financial Literacy for the Graduating Medical Student." *Med Educ* 45, no. 11 (2011): 1145–1146. https://doi.org/10.1111/j.1365-2923.2011.04131.x

6. Witek, M., J. Siglin, T. Malatesta, A. Snook, E. Gressen, S. Rudoler, V. Bar-Ad, and S. Fisher. "Is Financial Literacy Necessary for Radiation Oncology Residents?" *Int J Radiat Oncol Biol Phys* 90, no. 5 (2014): 986–987. https://doi.org/10.1016/j.ijrobp.2014.08.010

7. Merritt Hawkins. "2020 Review of Physician and Advanced Practitioner Recruiting Incentives and the Impact of COVID-19." 2020. https://www.merritthawkins.com/uploadedFiles/Merritt_Hawkins_Incentive_Review_2020.pdf.

8. Grayson, M.S., D.A. Newton, and L.F. Thompson. "Payback Time: The Associations of Debt and Income with Medical Student Career Choice." *Med Educ* 46, no. 10 (2012): 983–991. https://doi.org/10.1111/j.1365-2923.2012.04340.x

9. Morra, D.J., G. Regehr, and S. Ginsburg. "Medical Students, Money, and Career Selection: Students' Perception of Financial Factors and Remuneration in Family Medicine." *Fam Med* 41, no. 2 (2009): 105–110.

10. Rosenblatt, R.A., and C.H.A. Andrilla. "The Impact of U.S. Medical Students' Debt on Their Choice of Primary Care Careers: An Analysis of Data from

the 2002 Medical School Graduation Questionnaire." *Acad Med* 80, no. 9 (2005): 815–819. https://doi.org/10.1097/00001888-200509000-00006

11. Dall, T., and T. West. *The 2017 Update: Complexities of Physician Supply and Demand: Projections from 2015 to 2030.* Washington, DC: AAMC Workforce Study, 2017. https://doi.org/10.13140/RG.2.2.16013.95209

12. Esteves-Sorenson, C., and J. Snyder. "The Gender Earnings Gap for Physicians and Its Increase over Time." *Econ Lett* 116, no. 1 (2012): 37–41. https://doi.org/10.1016/j.econlet.2011.12.133

13. Frank, E., S.S. Zhuo Zhao, and C. Guille. "Gender Disparities in Work and Parental Status Among Early Career Physicians." *JAMA Network Open* 2, no. 8 (2019): e198340–e198340. https://doi.org/10.1001/jamanetworkopen.2019.8340

14. Association of American Medical Colleges. "Student Loan Repayment—Medical Schools and Students—Government Affairs—AAMC." https://students-residents.aamc.org/advocacy/article/student-debt/

15. Federal Student Aid. "Income-Driven Repayment Plans." https://studentaid.ed.gov/sa/repay-loans/understand/plans/income-driven

16. Dahle, J.M. *The White Coat Investor: A Doctor's Guide to Personal Finance and Investing.* White Coat Investor, 2014.

17. Kaiser Family Foundation. "Health Insurance Coverage of the Total Population." 2019. https://www.kff.org/other/state-indicator/total-population/

18. Ridic, G., S. Gleason, and O. Ridic. "Comparisons of Health Care systems in the United States, Germany and Canada." *Matera Sociomed* 24, no. 2 (2002): 112.

19. Terlizzi, E.P., R.A. Cohen, and M.E. Martinez. "Health Insurance Coverage: Early Release of Estimates from the National Health Interview Survey, January–September 2018." *Centers for Disease Control and Prevention.* February 2019. https://www.cdc.gov/nchs/data/nhis/earlyrelease/insur201902.pdf

20. Institute of Medicine and Committee on Enhancing Federal Healthcare Quality Programs. *Leadership by Example: Coordinating Government Roles in Improving Health Care Quality.* Edited by B.M. Smith, J. Eden, and J.M. Corrigan. Washington, DC: National Academies Press, 2003.

21. Papanicolas, I., L.R. Woskie, and A.K. Jha. "Health Care Spending in the United States and Other High-Income Countries." *JAMA* 319, no. 10 (2018): 1024–1039. https://doi.org/10.1001/jama.2018.1150

22. Davis, K., K. Stremikis, D. Squires, and C. Schoen. "Mirror, Mirror on the Wall." *The Commonwealth Fund.* June 2014. https://www.commonwealthfund.org/sites/default/files/documents/___media_files_publications_fund_report_2014_jun_1755_davis_mirror_mirror_2014.pdf

23. Berchick, E., J. Barnett, and R. Upton. "Health Insurance Coverage in the United States: 2018." *U.S. Census Bureau.* November 8, 2019. https://www.census.gov/library/publications/2019/demo/p60-267.html

24. The Patient Protection and Affordable Care Act (PPACA), Pub. L. No. 111-148, *124 Stat.* 119 (2010).

25. Bowling, B., D. Newman, C. White, A. Wood, and A. Coustasse. "Provider Reimbursement Following the Affordable Care Act." *Health Care Manag* 27, no. 2 (2018): 129–135. https://doi.org/10.1097/HCM.0000000000000205

26. Elsevier ClinicalKey. "How MACRA Will Affect Physicians in 2017." February 20, 2017. https://www.clinicalkey.com/info/blog/macra-will-affect-physicians-2017/

27. Guardado, J.R. "Medical Professional Liability Insurance Premiums: An Overview of the Market from 2009 to 2018." *American Medical Association.* January 2019. https://www.ama-assn.org/system/files/2019-01/policy-research-liability-premiums.pdf

28. Internal Revenue Service. "Types of Retirement Plans." September 22, 2020. https://www.irs.gov/retirement-plans/plan-sponsor/types-of-retirement-plans

15
The Aging Physician

Being a physician entails a process of lifelong learning and constant renewal of knowledge. Once working, physicians must maintain their credentials with yearly training and consistently review the relevant literature to stay up to date with current information and guidelines. However, due to many different factors, including financial pressures (see Chapter 14 of this volume), many physicians are continuing to work well into their 60s, 70s, and beyond. Many physicians may rightly feel that they have invested a significant amount of time into being a physician and, as a result, continue to practice as they advance in age. Many physicians love their work and laudably view it as part of their identity rather than a job. Why think about retirement if you are following a calling to do what you love every day?

These trends have contributed to the "graying" of the American physician population. In 2015, 23 percent of American physicians were older than 65 years old, representing nearly a 400 percent increase from 1975.[1] Some specialties are disproportionately older, particularly in primary care; for example, 89 percent of physicians specializing in pulmonary disease were 55 years or older. Additionally, these numbers are expected to increase in the future. The physician population continues to age, and many physicians continue to work past the traditional retirement age of 65. This may seem innocuous, and possibly even good, at first glance. As the rest of the American population ages and the strain on the healthcare system increases, wouldn't it be good to have more doctors, especially those who are more experienced? While this may be partially true, the aging of the physician workforce brings up concerns about physician shortages, particularly in primary care, in which demand continues to increase as the general population ages.

Aging physicians may also present some danger to their patients due to the effects of cognitive decline. Some aspects of cognitive decline may be seen as a natural part of aging, but in a profession in which cognitive ability has the potential to affect patient safety, it is of utmost importance that guidelines exist for evaluating aging physicians. Furthermore, mild cognitive impairment (MCI) represents a state of cognitive decline that is greater than that of normal aging[2] and is estimated to be present in 10 to 20 percent of people aged 65 and older.[3] The math suggests that about 25,000 to 50,000 physicians over the age of 65 with cognitive impairment are involved in active patient care. These figures are supported by the evidence: a study found that there is a decline in psychomotor and visuospatial skills in aging surgeons.[4] However, the changes due to MCI are often subtle, and physicians may not realize that they are impaired. Nevertheless, they may put their patients in danger by continuing to practice. Research shows that surgeons over the age of 60 have higher mortality outcomes in complex procedures.[5] Medicare patients treated by older physicians were found to have higher mortality rates within 30 days of hospitalization.[6] A systematic review of the literature found that there may be an inverse relationship between the number of years that a physician has been in practice and the quality of care that they provide.[7]

There are also concerns associated with dementia and other serious cognitive disorders associated with aging. Approximately 10 percent of Americans above the age of 65 are estimated to suffer from Alzheimer's dementia.[8] Extrapolating from the number of physicians above the age of 65, if physicians suffer from dementia at similar rates as the general population, there are approximately 25,000 currently practicing physicians with dementia. We would like to believe that physicians are at lower risk than the general population for dementia due to healthy lifestyle habits, but there are likely still a significant number of physicians who have dementia.[9]

These statistics bring up many questions: How exactly does aging lead to cognitive decline? How do we prevent those who are no longer capable of caring for patients from inadvertently causing harm? And how do we do so in a way that maintains the dignity of all older physicians?

Cognitive changes due to aging

Cognitive changes due to aging can be classified as normal or abnormal. A growing amount of evidence suggests that normal cognitive decline is distinct from MCI, which is further distinct from impairment due to dementia. Normal cognitive changes include a steady decline in certain cognitive functions, which generally does not have much effect on day-to-day life. On the other end of the spectrum, severe impairment due to Alzheimer's dementia may lead to significant problems with memory loss and behavior.

Normal cognitive changes due to aging

Crystallized intelligence, which describes accumulated knowledge and expertise, is largely resistant to cognitive decline.[10] On the other hand, *fluid intelligence*, which is implicated in problem-solving and reasoning about things that are less familiar or unlearned, tends to decline after a peak during the third decade of life.[11] Processes implicated in fluid intelligence include analytic processing, reaction time, fine motor skill, dexterity, learning, comprehension, and attention. Therefore, while certain cognitive functions may be stable or improve with age, others may decrease (see Figure 15.1).

Processing speed refers to the speed at which cognitive processes are performed, as well as the speed of motor responses. As an element of fluid intelligence, it tends to decline with age. In fact, many of the normal cognitive changes associated with aging may be the result of slowed processing speed.[12] Declines in processing speed may have detrimental effects across many different cognitive domains, including attention, memory, and executive functioning.

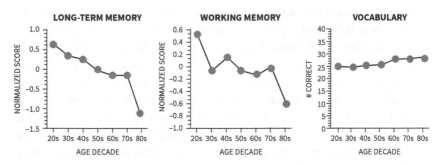

Figure 15.1 Aging preferentially influences some cognitive domains more than others.

From Randy L. Buckner, "Memory and Executive Function in Aging and AD: Multiple Factors That Cause Decline and Reserve Factors That Compensate." *Neuron* 44, no. 1 (September 30, 2004): 196, Figure 2, with permission from Elsevier.

Attention, or the ability to concentrate and focus on specific stimuli, is another fluid intelligence construct that tends to decline with age. While there are no differences observed due to aging in simple attention tasks, such as the digit-span memory test, performance tends to decrease in complex attention tasks involving selective or divided attention[10] Selective attention refers to the ability to focus on specific information in an environment while filtering out irrelevant information. Divided attention refers to the ability to focus on multiple tasks simultaneously.

Memory is another cognitive construct that may be affected by aging. While some types of memory—such as sensory, episodic, and procedural memory—tend to be stable with age, other types of memory—such as source, working, and prospective memory—tend to decline with age.

Executive functioning refers to the collection of mental processes necessary when one must concentrate and pay attention to complete a task, when relying on instinct is ill-advised or impossible.[13] It is generally agreed that there are three core executive functions: inhibition and interference control, working memory, and cognitive flexibility. From these, higher-order executive functions such as reasoning, problem-solving, and planning may be built.[14] Research suggests that many of these functions decline with age.[15] Older individuals tend to think more concretely, and abstraction and mental flexibility decline with age.[16] Inductive reasoning ability also tends to decline normally with age, as well as the ability to reason about unfamiliar material.[17]

Based on the normal cognitive changes due to aging, it seems likely that while most aging physicians may still be able to execute their old, mastered techniques, some may struggle to complete complex analytical tasks or develop new skills. Older physicians may rely more heavily on nonanalytic reasoning and use the knowledge base they have developed over their careers. This is not necessarily a bad thing; studies suggest that older physicians make more accurate initial diagnoses for this very reason.[18] However, when conflicting or new information is provided, nonanalytic reasoning may be insufficient. Furthermore, many of the tasks that physicians are required to perform require skills attributable to fluid intelligence constructs. For example, a surgeon will likely need to use selective attention and mental flexibility to perform a difficult operation.

It is important to note that aging does not lead to declines in cognitive performance for all physicians, however. Although average cognitive performance tends to be lower for older physicians, many older physicians perform

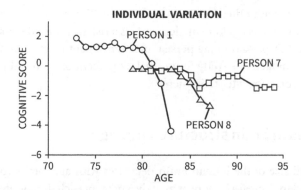

Figure 15.2 Individual variation in cognitive function associated with aging.
From Randy L. Buckner, "Memory and Executive Function in Aging and AD: Multiple Factors That Cause Decline and Reserve Factors That Compensate." *Neuron* 44, no. 1 (September 30, 2004): 196, Figure 1, with permission from Elsevier.

at an equal or higher level than their younger colleagues.[19] Longitudinal studies show that the individual variability of cognitive performance increases with age.[20] Both genetic and environmental factors contribute to the degree of decline, and decline in cognitive function with age is highly variable among individuals.[21] Figure 15.2 shows the individual variation in cognitive function associated with age.

Dementia and Alzheimer's disease

In addition to the normal cognitive declines associated with aging, there are also serious mental health conditions associated with old age. It is estimated that 10 percent of Americans over the age of 65 suffer from Alzheimer's dementia.[8] MCI may, at times, represent an early stage of Alzheimer's disease, which may progress to dementia later on. In the later stages of dementia, significant decreases in cognitive function may arise, including symptoms such as memory loss or confusion regarding time and place, as well as behavioral symptoms such as depression and personality changes.

It is estimated that 20 percent of people ages 55 and older experience some kind of mental health issue.[22] Incidence of depression and rates of suicide increase with age, but symptoms are often overlooked and untreated because they coincide with other medical conditions or life events.[23] Although the exact relationship is not known, dementia is a risk factor for depression, and vice versa.[24] Depression may persist after retirement or even as a result of retirement. In fact, one study found that 27 percent of surveyed physicians reported depression after retirement.[25]

Changes in brain structure with age

The overall size of the human brain decreases with age. Brain volume has been found to decrease by approximately 5 percent each decade after the age of 40.[26] Within the past 20 years or so, the use of magnetic resonance imaging and computed tomography have allowed us to better understand this atrophy. Both gray and white manner volume decrease with age. However, regions of the brain have been found to atrophy at different rates. The greatest gray matter loss is found in the prefrontal cortex, a region of the brain implicated in complex decision-making.[26] Gray matter volume also decreases in the temporal lobes, including the hippocampus, which has important functions for learning and memory.[27] Significant white matter decreases have been observed in the frontal lobe and regions of high white matter density such as the corpus callosum.[28] These structural changes in the brain are in line with the functional changes observed due to cognitive aging.

Guidelines for evaluating aging physicians

Clearly, there needs to be a system for identifying when physicians can no longer provide adequate care to their patients. But what is fair? Should there be a mandatory retirement age? Should there be required mental and physical screening after some age? Who should oversee these efforts? Should they be individual practices, hospitals, state licensing boards, or state and federal law? These questions are fraught with difficulties.

While an amendment to the Age Discrimination in Employment Act in 1986 outlawed mandatory retirement based on age,[29] Congress and state governments mandate retirement ages for certain high-reliability professions that may impact public safety (see Table 15.1).[30–32] However, as of now, there are no such requirements in the medical profession.

Table 15.1 Professions with Mandatory Retirement Ages

Profession	Mandated Age of Retirement	Other Special Considerations
Commercial Airline Pilot	65	Screenings beginning at the age of 40
Federal Law Enforcement Officer (FBI Special Agent, National Park Ranger, Custom/Border Protection Officer, Lighthouse Operator)	57	Exemptions granted by departmental agency heads when in the public interest; may work past mandatory retirement age if 20 years of service have not been accumulated
Nuclear Weapons Courier	57	
Firefighter	57	
Air Traffic Controller	56	
State Judge	70–75	Depends on the state, but as of now, most states have a mandatory retirement age for judges between 70 and 75. For example, in New York, judges must retire by 70.

In certain states, it may be easier to renew a medical license than to maintain a driver's license. For example, in Illinois, citizens above the age of 75 are required to take a road test to determine driving competency.[33] On the other hand, while Illinois medical licenses must be renewed every three years, after the initial exam, no competency-based tests are required.[34]

Currently, the system in place for evaluating physicians who are impaired due to aging is one of self-regulation.[35] Physicians are expected to report themselves or their colleagues when they believe that they are impaired, as per the American Medical Association's (AMA) Code of Medical Ethics.[36] But there are many obstacles to overcome before this can come to fruition (see Chapter 12 of this volume):

- Physicians must identify that they or their colleague is impaired, which can often be quite challenging. Studies have shown that physicians possess a limited ability to assess their own competence and cognitive decline.[37]

- Because physicians are generally high-functioning and resourceful, they may be able to compensate for their MCI by avoiding certain procedures, using extra help from their peers or support staff, or taking fewer patients. There are many strategies that physicians may utilize to hide their cognitive impairment from their peers, similar to how physicians suffering from mental health disorders or substance use disorders may effectively hide their conditions (see Chapters 11 and 12 of this volume).
- Once impairment due to cognitive decline is identified, it may be difficult to report due to stigma as well as professional and social pressures. One study found that physicians would be more likely to report a colleague impaired due to substance use compared to one suffering from cognitive decline or psychological impairment.[38] Reporting senior practitioners—who are often the most respected members of the community and who may have served as teachers and mentors—may be incredibly challenging for many physicians.

Recently, there has been a push for cognitive screening as part of the credentialing process for physicians above the age of 65 to ensure fitness for duty. In 2015, the AMA Council on Medical Education issued a report calling for the establishment of guidelines for assessing the competency of aging physicians.[39] Many hospitals and academic institutions have begun to develop their own policies to address these concerns. For example, Stanford requires a multicomponent screening process for physicians above the age of 75 to be completed every two years.[40] Yale New Haven Hospital requires neurologic and ophthalmologic exams for physicians above the age of 70; it found that between 2016 and 2019, 12.7 percent of the physicians tested demonstrated cognitive deficits that were likely to impair their ability to practice.[41]

However, even though these policies have been established with patient safety in mind and while it is evident that current policies of self-regulation are insufficient, these screening policies have largely been met with controversy and pushback. For example, a group of physicians at Stanford successfully lobbied to remove the cognitive component of their program for assessing aging physicians.[42] Opposition by the Utah Medical Association led to the passage of a state law banning age-based physician screening.[43]

Many older physicians do not want or cannot afford to retire, and screening programs are, in general, difficult to implement. Because prevalence of the condition is low, there are likely to be false-positives unless the test has very high specificity. False-positive results are likely to be highly detrimental, as they may affect the careers of practicing physicians. In addition, assessing clinical competence is not an exact science, and screening for high-risk groups may be legally and socially problematic. A report published by California Public Protection and Physician Health in 2015 examines the legal issues of screening aging physicians.[44]

The optimal solution is likely to be multipronged and multifactorial, requiring coordination with state medical boards as well as an individualized multistep evaluation process. One suggested element is a screening process that incorporates a highly sensitive initial test, followed by higher-specificity assessments for those who screen positive.[45] Incorporating multiple sources, including clinical documentation, board certification information, peer assessments, and simulation testing may also be useful. Furthermore, policies that encourage successful aging and protect against cognitive decline in physicians are likely to be effective in protecting patient safety. A policy that balances patient safety with the dignity of aging physicians is likely to be most effective.

Successful aging and adjustment to retirement

Growing evidence suggests that healthy lifestyle practices may protect against age-related cognitive decline. For example, one study showed that physical activity may improve cognition and protect against MCI and dementia.[46] On the other hand, systemic inflammation during midlife was associated with decreased late-life brain volume.[47] A lack of social support is also associated with a decline in cognitive function.[48] Sleep dysfunctions have been found to be associated with Alzheimer's dementia.[49] Therefore, adoption of a variety of practices in lifestyle medicine throughout one's career may allow for successful aging (see Chapter 9 of this volume).

Many aging physicians may be reluctant to retire. Many fear that they will lose part of their core identity and life purpose.[50] Financial concerns also play a significant role (see Chapter 14 of this volume). It is important to identify the needs of physicians and the factors that allow for successful adjustment to retirement. The key factors for physicians' adjustment to retirement have been identified as financial security, favorable health, engagement in activities, and psychosocial well-being. Therefore, it seems prudent to provide medical professionals with adequate resources for developing financial literacy (see Chapter 14 of this volume) and lifestyle practices for maintaining their physical and mental health (see Chapter 9 of this volume). Not only will these be vital for maintaining well-being during physicians' years of practice but will also benefit them when they age and plan to retire.

Many physicians are reluctant to give up all engagement with medicine when they retire, underscoring that the medical profession is a calling for many, rather than just a job. This suggests that the transition to retirement may also be eased by providing opportunities for aging physicians to continue in mentorship roles or research.[51] For example, Michael DeBakey, a renowned cardiovascular surgeon and pioneer of the cardiopulmonary bypass surgery, ceased operating in his later years but continued to maintain an active schedule of lecturing and teaching until his death at the age of 99. Shigeaki Hinohara, who is often credited with building the foundation for modern Japanese medicine, published numerous books in his later life until his death at the age of 105. By continuing to support physicians' engagement with the medical profession, even after retirement, we may be able to respect their dignity and ease the often-difficult transition process.

Chapter Quick Summary

- There is a "graying" of the American physician workforce.
- In addition to concerns about physician shortages once aging physicians retire, there are also significant concerns about patient safety due to physicians' cognitive decline from aging.
- Normal cognitive changes due to aging include a decline in fluid intelligence domains, such as processing speed, complex attention, working memory, and executive functioning.
- Dementia from Alzheimer's disease, as well as other mental health conditions, may lead to abnormal cognitive changes that cause impairment.
- The current system of self-regulation to identify physicians who are impaired due to cognitive decline is likely to be insufficient for

protecting patient safety; on the other hand, mandatory retirement or screening of aging physicians may be ethically or legally problematic.

- Adoption of healthy lifestyle practices and financial literacy may encourage successful aging and ease the transition to retirement.
- Providing opportunities for retired physicians to stay involved with the medical profession may also prove valuable.

Resources

Alzheimer's Association. "Alzheimer's and Dementia." https://www.alz.org/alzheimer_s_dementia

American Medical Association. "Retire and Stay Active Within the Medical Community." https://www.ama-assn.org/practice-management/career-development/retire-and-stay-active-within-medical-community

California Public Protection and Physician Health, Inc. "Assessing Late Career Practitioners: Policies and Procedures for Age-Based Screening." July 2015. https://www.cppph.org/wp-content/uploads/2015/07/assessing-late-career-practitioners-adopted-by-cppph-changes-6-10-151.pdf

National Institute on Aging. [Home page]. https://www.nia.nih.gov/

References

1. American Medical Association. *Competency and the Aging Physician. Report 5 of the Council on Medical Education (A-15).* Chicago, IL: AMA, 2015.
2. Petersen, R.C. "Mild Cognitive Impairment." *Continuum* 22, no. 2 (2016): 404–418. https://doi.org/10.1212/CON.0000000000000313
3. Langa, K.M., and D.A. Levine. "The Diagnosis and Management of Mild Cognitive Impairment: A Clinical Review." *JAMA* 312, no. 23 (2014): 2551–2561. https://doi.org/10.1001/jama.2014.13806
4. Boom-Saad, Z., S.A. Langenecker, L.A. Bieliauskas, C.J. Graver, J.R. O'Neill, A.F. Caveney, L.J. Greenfield, and R.M. Minter. "Surgeons Outperform Normative Controls on Neuropsychologic Tests, but Age-Related Decay of Skills Persists." *Am J Surg* 195, no. 2 (February 2008): 205–209. https://doi.org/10.1016/j.amjsurg.2007.11.002

5. Waljee, J.F., L.J. Greenfield, J.B. Dimick, and J.D. Birkmeyer. "Surgeon Age and Operative Mortality in the United States." *Ann Surg* 244, no. 3 (September 2006): 353–362. https://doi.org/10.1097/01.sla.0000234803.11991.6d

6. Tsugawa, Y., J.P. Newhouse, A.M. Zaslavsky, D.M. Blumenthal, and A.B. Jena. "Physician Age and Outcomes in Elderly Patients in Hospital in the US: Observational Study." *BMJ* 357 (2017):j1797. https://doi.org/10.1136/bmj.j1797

7. Choudhry, N.K., R.H. Fletcher, and S.B. Soumerai. "Systematic Review: The Relationship between Clinical Experience and Quality of Health Care." *Ann Inter Med* 142, no. 4 (2005): 260–273. https://doi.org/10.7326/0003-4819-142-4-200502150-00008

8. "2020 Alzheimer's Disease Facts and Figures." *Alzheimer's & Dementia* 16, no. 3 (2020): 391–460. https://doi.org/10.1002/alz.12068

9. Sabayan, B., and F. Sorond. "Reducing Risk of Dementia in Older Age." *JAMA* 317, no. 19 (2017): 2028. https://doi.org/10.1001/jama.2017.2247

10. Lezak, M., D. Howieson, E. Bigler, and D. Tranel. *Neuropsychological Assessment.* 5th ed. Oxford: Oxford University Press, 2012.

11. Salthouse, T. "Consequences of Age-Related Cognitive Declines." *Ann Rev Psychol* 63 (2012): 201–226. https://doi.org/10.1146/annurev-psych-120710-100328

12. Harada, C.N., M.C. Natelson Love, and K. Triebel. "Normal Cognitive Aging." *Clin Geriatr Med* 29, no. 4 (November 2013): 737–752. https://doi.org/10.1016/j.cger.2013.07.002.

13. Diamond, A. "Executive Functions." *Ann Rev Psychol* 64 (2013): 135–168. https://doi.org/10.1146/annurev-psych-113011-143750

14. Collins, A., and E. Koechlin. "Reasoning, Learning, and Creativity: Frontal Lobe Function and Human Decision-Making." *PLOS Biology* 10, no. 3 (2012): e1001293. https://doi.org/10.1371/journal.pbio.1001293

15. Salthouse, T.A. "Selective Review of Cognitive Aging." *JINS* 16, no. 5 2010): 754–760. https://doi.org/10.1017/S1355617710000706

16. Oosterman, J.M., R.L.C. Vogels, B. van Harten, A.A. Gouw, A. Poggesi, P. Scheltens, R.P.C. Kessels, and E.J.A. Scherder. "Assessing Mental Flexibility: Neuroanatomical and Neuropsychological Correlates of the Trail Making Test in Elderly People." *Clin Neuropsychol* 24, no. 2 (2010): 203–219. https://doi.org/10.1080/13854040903482848

17. Singh-Manoux, A., M. Kivimaki, M.M. Glymour, A. Elbaz, C. Berr, K.P. Ebmeier, J.E. Ferrie, and A. Dugravot. "Timing of Onset of Cognitive Decline: Results

from Whitehall II Prospective Cohort Study." *BMJ* 344 (2012), https://doi.org/10.1136/bmj.d7622

18. Hobus, P.P., H.G. Schmidt, H.P. Boshuizen, and V.L. Patel. "Contextual Factors in the Activation of First Diagnostic Hypotheses: Expert-Novice Differences." *Med Educ* 21, no. 6 (1987): 471–476. https://doi.org/10.1111/j.1365-2923.1987.tb01405.x

19. Drag, L.L., L.A Bieliauskas, S.A Langenecker, and L.J Greenfield. "Cognitive Functioning, Retirement Status, and Age: Results from the Cognitive Changes and Retirement among Senior Surgeons Study." *J Am Coll Surg* 211, no. 3 (2010): 303–307. https://doi.org/10.1016/j.jamcollsurg.2010.05.022

20. Small, B.J., R.A. Dixon, and J.J. McArdle. "Tracking Cognition–Health Changes From 55 to 95 Years of Age." *J Gerontol B-Psychol* 66B, no. Suppl 1 (2011): i153–i161. https://doi.org/10.1093/geronb/gbq093

21. Deary, I.J., J. Yang, G. Davies, S.E. Harris, A. Tenesa, D. Liewald, M. Luciano, L.M. Lopez, A.J. Gow, J. Corley, P. Redmond, H.C. Fox, S.J. Rowe, P. Haggarty, G. McNeill, M.E. Goddard, D.J. Porteous, L.J. Whalley, J.M. Starr, and P.M. Visscher. "Genetic Contributions to Stability and Change in Intelligence from Childhood to Old Age." *Nature* 481, no. 7384 (2012): 212–215. https://doi.org/10.1038/nature10781

22. American Psychiatric Association. "Growing Mental and Behavioral Health Concerns Facing Older Americans." August 2018. https://www.apa.org/advocacy/health/older-americans-mental-behavioral-health

23. Rodda, J., Z. Walker, and J. Carter. "Depression in Older Adults." *BMJ* 343 (2011). https://doi.org/10.1136/bmj.d5219

24. Rubin, R. "Exploring the Relationship Between Depression and Dementia." *JAMA* 320, no. 10 (2018): 961–962. https://doi.org/10.1001/jama.2018.11154

25. Lees, E., S.E. Liss, I.M. Cohen, J.N. Kvale, and S.K. Ostwald. "Emotional Impact of Retirement on Physicians." *Texas Med* 97, no. 9 (2001): 66–71.

26. Svennerholm, L., K. Boström, and B. Jungbjer. "Changes in Weight and Compositions of Major Membrane Components of Human Brain during the Span of Adult Human Life of Swedes." *Acta Neuropathol* 94, no. 4 (October 1997): 345–352. https://doi.org/10.1007/s004010050717

27. Scahill, R.I., C. Frost, R. Jenkins, J.L. Whitwell, M.N. Rossor, and N.C. Fox. "A Longitudinal Study of Brain Volume Changes in Normal Aging Using Serial Registered Magnetic Resonance Imaging." *Arch Neurol* 60, no. 7 (July 2003): 989–994. https://doi.org/10.1001/archneur.60.7.989

28. Salat, D.H., J.A. Kaye, and J.S. Janowsky. "Prefrontal Gray and White Matter Volumes in Healthy Aging and Alzheimer Disease." *Arch Neurol* 56, no. 3 (March 1999): 338–344. https://doi.org/10.1001/archneur.56.3.338

29. Age Discrimination in Employment Act of 1967 (Pub. L. 90-202) (1967). https://www.eeoc.gov/statutes/age-discrimination-employment-act-1967

30. Aviation Pros. "FAA to Propose Pilot Retirement Age Change." January 30, 2007. https://www.aviationpros.com/home/press-release/10433304/faa-to-propose-pilot-retirement-age-change

31. "20 Year Retirement Eligibility: LEO, FF, ATC & NWC Annuity Calculations." June 10, 2020. *Federal Retirement Planning.* https://www.federalretirement.net/eligibility20years.htm#Mandatory_Separations

32. "Mandatory Retirement." *Ballotpedia.* https://ballotpedia.org/Mandatory_retirement

33. Repa, B.K. "Illinois Driving Laws for Seniors and Older Drivers." *Nolo.* Updated by V. Keene. https://www.nolo.com/legal-encyclopedia/illinois-driving-laws-seniors-older-drivers.html.

34. Illinois State Medical Association. "Illinois State Medical Society Medical Licensure and CME Information." 2020. https://www.isms.org/Resources/For_Physicians/Licensure_and_Credentialing/Medical_Licensure_and_CME_Information/

35. Wynia, M.K. "The Role of Professionalism and Self-Regulation in Detecting Impaired or Incompetent Physicians." *JAMA* 304, no. 2 (2010): 210–212. https://doi.org/10.1001/jama.2010.945

36. American Medical Association. "AMA Code of Medical Ethics Opinion 9.3.2 Physician Responsibilities to Impaired Colleagues." https://www.ama-assn.org/delivering-care/ethics/physician-responsibilities-impaired-colleagues

37. Davis, D.A., P.E. Mazmanian, M. Fordis, R. Van Harrison, K.E. Thorpe, and L. Perrier. "Accuracy of Physician Self-Assessment Compared with Observed Measures of Competence: A Systematic Review." *JAMA* 296, no. 9 (2006): 1094–1102. https://doi.org/10.1001/jama.296.9.1094

38. Farber, N.J., S.G. Gilibert, B.M. Aboff, V.U. Collier, J. Weiner, and E.G. Boyer. "Physicians' Willingness to Report Impaired Colleagues." *Soc Sci Med* 61, no. 8 (2005): 1772–1775. https://doi.org/10.1016/j.socscimed.2005.03.029

39. AMA Council on Medical Education. "Report 5 of the Council on Medical Education (A-15) Competency and the Aging Physician." *California Public Protection & Physician Health.* February 2016. https://www.cppph.org/wp-content/uploads/2016/02/AMA-Council-on-Medical-Education-Aging-Physician-Report-2015.pdf

40. Stanford Health Care. "Stanford to Implement a Late Career Practitioner Policy." August 2012. https://stanfordhealthcare.org/health-care-professionals/medical-staff/medstaff-update/2012-august/stanford-to-implement-a-late-career-practitioner-policy.html

41. Cooney, L., and T. Balcezak. "Cognitive Testing of Older Clinicians Prior to Recredentialing." *JAMA* 323, no. 2 (2020): 179–180. https://doi.org/10.1001/jama.2019.18665

42. Krieger, L.M. "Stanford Doctors Fight Age-Related Test of Fitness to Practice." *The Mercury News (San Jose)*. June 8, 2015. http://www.mercurynews.com/2015/06/08/Stanford-doctors-fight-age-related-test-of-fitness-to-practice

43. Physician Testing Amendments, SB 217, UT Gen Sess (2018).

44. California Public Protection and Physician Health, Inc. "Assessing Late Career Practitioners: Policies and Procedures for Age-Based Screening." July 2015. https://www.cppph.org/wp-content/uploads/2015/07/assessing-late-career-practitioners-adopted-by-cppph-changes-6-10-151.pdf

45. Armstrong, K.A., and E.E. Reynolds. "Opportunities and Challenges in Valuing and Evaluating Aging Physicians." *JAMA* 323, no. 2 (2020): 125–126. https://doi.org/10.1001/jama.2019.19706

46. Nuzum, H., A. Stickel, M. Corona, M. Zeller, R.J. Melrose, and S.S. Wilkins. "Potential Benefits of Physical Activity in MCI and Dementia." *Behav Neurol* 2020 (2020): 7807856. https://doi.org/10.1155/2020/7807856

47. Walker, K.A., R.F. Gottesman, A. Wu, D.S. Knopman, A.L. Gross, T.H. Mosley, E. Selvin, and B.G. Windham. "Systemic Inflammation during Midlife and Cognitive Change over 20 Years: The ARIC Study." *Neurol* 92, no. 11 (2019): e1256–e1267. https://doi.org/10.1212/WNL.0000000000007094

48. Donovan, N.J., Q. Wu, D.M. Rentz, R.A. Sperling, G.A. Marshall, and M.M. Glymour. "Loneliness, Depression and Cognitive Function in Older U.S. Adults." *Int J Geriatr Psychiatr* 32, no. 5 (May 2017): 564–573. https://doi.org/10.1002/gps.4495

49. Proserpio, P., D. Arnaldi, F. Nobili, and L. Nobili. "Integrating Sleep and Alzheimer's Disease Pathophysiology: Hints for Sleep Disorders Management." *JAD* 63, no. 3 (2018): 871–86. https://doi.org/10.3233/JAD-180041

50. Silver, M.P., N.C. Pang, and S.A. Williams. "'Why Give Up Something That Works So Well?' Retirement Expectations Among Academic Physicians." *Educ Gerontol* 41, no. 5 (May 4, 2015): 333–347. https://doi.org/10.1080/03601277.2014.970419

51. Jeste, D.V., and T.T. Nguyen. "Successful Aging of Physicians." *Am J Geriatr Psychiatr* 26, no. 2 (2018): 209–211. https://doi.org/10.1016/j.jagp.2017.08.003

16
Looking to the Future

The physician's role is continually changing and is sure to undergo significant changes in the near future. For those of us who have spent many sleepless nights memorizing concepts, learning skills, and integrating complex medical decision-making processes into our professional cognitive processes (or clinical skills and armamentarium), we may think, "Why do we have to constantly modify our foundational knowledge?" Consider the rate at which medical knowledge has increased. It has been estimated that the doubling time of medical knowledge in 1950 was 50 years; in 1980, 7 years; and in 2010, 3.5 years. An oft-cited estimate for the doubling time of medical knowledge in 2020 is 73 days.[1] While this figure may not be accurate, it stands that the volume of medical knowledge continues to increase at a faster and faster rate. With this in mind, the necessity of the professional mandate for lifelong learning and constant renewal of knowledge and skills is quite evident.

The responsibilities of the medical profession have changed dramatically in the past and will continue to do so in the future. Consider the role of religion in medicine and how it has continued to evolve over the past two or three centuries. Western medicine has undergone a shift away from religion, and during this transition period, physicians' responsibilities regarding the balance of clinical and spiritual care have been blurred. Even now, it is often confusing what the professional and ethical boundaries are regarding religion and spirituality in our practices. While the historical role of the physician as a spiritual healer has largely diminished, physicians would be well-served to understand that religion and spirituality play in important role in healthcare.

There are many factors currently at play in the current healthcare environment that will lead to significant changes in our responsibilities as physicians. In particular, the COVID-19 pandemic is likely to be an important turning point for the medical profession. While the pandemic has shown the remarkable resilience of physicians across the globe, this level of engagement was generated out of necessity. After the pandemic is over, we suspect that physicians will suffer from greater degrees of disengagement and burnout than ever before; we will deal with the impact of what was originally described by Tseng as the fourth wave of the COVID-19 pandemic—which has subsequently been called the fifth wave—referring to the long-term mental trauma associated with dealing with the disease.[2]

This fifth wave will continue rising over the next several years. In addition, it will affect each of the previous waves: the first wave, which refers to the immediate morbidity and mortality associated with COVID-19; the second wave, which refers to the morbidity and mortality from other diseases due to resource restrictions imposed by the pandemic; the third wave, which refers to the impact multiple future waves of COVID-19 infection as stay-at-home orders are relaxed; and the fourth wave, which refers to the impact of interrupted care for chronic conditions.

While the COVID-19 pandemic has certainly highlighted the professionalism and leadership of physicians across the world, it has put undue stress on members of our community as well. One preliminary study reported troubling results regarding mental health outcomes for healthcare providers involved in treating coronavirus disease: 50.4 percent had symptoms of depression, 34.0 percent reported insomnia, 44.6 percent reported symptoms of anxiety, and 71.5 percent reported distress.[3] The pandemic has brought to light many of the issues that physicians face today, and we hope that it will serve as a wake-up call to address physician burnout and promote physician well-being. We must work as a community to combat the underlying factors contributing to burnout, not just as a responsibility to ourselves, but to our patients as well.

The unsustainable burden of treating chronic conditions will likely also lead to changes in our roles as physicians, particularly as the global population continues to age—it is estimated that over the next 30 years that the population over 65 will be twice that of the population below 5 years old. We must develop ways to address the burden of aging and chronic disease. Much of the current focus in healthcare is on treating disease rather than preventing it. Many have recognized that this model is flawed. Indeed, the COVID-19 pandemic has highlighted the increased risk of serious illness associated with underlying chronic conditions.[4] In the near future, we must work to better understand the mechanisms of innate and adaptive immunity and espouse the value of prevention through lifestyle (see Chapter 9). We need healthcare systems to be incentivized to give physicians enough time with patients to address chronic diseases and mental health concerns. We require policies that allow physicians support, education, and resources to engage with patients at an individual level and communicate appropriate interventions to prevent disease, disability, and death.

The process of lifelong learning entails that physicians are committed to continually improve our knowledge and skills to deliver a high standard of care. However, self-regulation, the process that underlies lifelong learning, is unable to be employed when physicians are afflicted with feelings of disengagement and depersonalization due to burnout.[5] As stressed throughout the book, our well-being is important to patient care. Many of us in the profession have a well-intentioned belief that sacrificing our well-being for more time with patients is good or even necessary, but, in fact, this goes against our commitment to professionalism.

Physicians are healers, lifelong learners, and teachers, but many are also employees. In the past, nearly all physicians were in charge of their own practices and had significant amount of control over hospital operations. Now, the number of physicians who are employed exceeds those who own their own practices, and the trend toward employment is likely to accelerate after COVID-19.[6] Healthcare is changing, and our roles as physicians are increasingly being defined by externalities such as insurance companies, pharmaceutical makers, and administrators. The *consumerization* of medicine has at times challenged physicians' ethical imperative to put patient well-being first: as employees, physicians must balance their fiduciary duty to the patient with their duty to the employer. For example, physicians may be pressured to reduce costs by spending less time with patients, which may be in direct conflict with their moral responsibility to care for patients. This is a concept called *moral distress*. Moral distress may result from power imbalances between members of the healthcare team, patient or family preferences, poor communication, pressure to reduce costs, fear of legal action, lack of administrative support, or hospital policies that may conflict with patient care needs.[7] Moral distress may lead to alienation, detachment, and loss of empathy and may contribute to burnout. We believe that physicians not being engaged in the decision-making process may have contributed to many of the issues in dealing with the COVID-19 pandemic. For example, decisions to admit patients and ration personal protective equipment were often made without consulting physicians. Restoring physician autonomy may be valuable for all those involved in healthcare.

The adoption of new technologies and policies will also serve as disruptions to the profession. How exactly will our roles change? And how can we position ourselves to adapt to these changes? With the shift toward employment and the advent of electronic health records, many physicians are finding challenges in engaging with patients.[8] Many are disengaged or suffering from burnout. As a result, their ability to connect empathically with patients may suffer. Further incorporation of new digital technologies may lead to novel challenges in communication within the profession. Even now, younger physicians who grew up with social media and use it as a primary means of communication may experience a divide with older physicians who are unfamiliar with the technology. This is only the tip of the iceberg for how technology will transform the profession. However, these changes ought not to worry us, as they are a natural part of the evolution of healthcare and society.

Consider this: when the phone was invented, the generation that did not grow up with this technology was in uproar about how it would ruin all social interactions; they insisted that the only way to communicate for respectable members of society was in person. When social media was created, a bill in 2006 was introduced in the House of Representatives entitled the Deleting Online Predators Act to outlaw it in schools and libraries.[9] Although this bill did not pass, it highlights the fear that was associated with the advent of social media. Although there are still people who do not like it and do not engage in online communication, the majority of us do.

During the COVID-19 crisis, telehealth, or telemedicine, has overnight become an acceptable means of physician–patient communication. Telehealth is an exciting way in which technology has begun to be used in modern medicine as a force multiplier for medical training, communication, and collaboration. Defined as "the use of electronic information and communications technology to provide and support healthcare when distance separates the participants," telehealth allows for the sharing of more varied and specialized knowledge required in the rapidly expanding field of medicine. Still, the use of telehealth may be more effective for certain types of knowledge transfer than others. Telehealth projects involving the communication of tacit knowledge, defined as knowledge that cannot be easily written down and that "has a personal component that makes it difficult to communicate to others in an understandable form," may have more positive results than teleconsultation and distance-learning projects that involve primarily the transfer of explicit knowledge.[10p144]

While telehealth is not new, widespread adoption by healthcare providers has been slow. However, recently, because of the COVID-19 pandemic, barriers to telehealth access have been significantly reduced, and telehealth has arisen as a way to deliver acute, chronic, primary, and specialty care. Telehealth has incredible potential for both training and delivering care in low-income and rural regions. Technological advancements have also rendered international borders more fluid, allowing for medical interactions that extend past traditional boundaries. In doing so, telehealth may serve as an enabler for value-based care.

There are some issues with telehealth that must be addressed. For example, licensure and regulation may vary by state, and issues may arise if a clinician conducts a patient interview across state lines. Some situations may not be possible to address without the ability to perform an in-person physical exam. Patients may have concerns about privacy, and patients or physicians may struggle with the technology. Patients and clinicians alike may not have the resources to support telehealth technologies. However, over time, as telehealth becomes more widespread, these issues are likely to be resolved, paving the way for telehealth to be used to deliver better care. Even now, federal regulations on telehealth have begun to be relaxed, and Medicare has recently expanded coverage for telehealth. As physician–patient interactions increasingly enter the online space, our roles may certainly change. However, it is likely that our ability to communicate empathically with patients will remain our most valuable value-add.

Another way in which technology will soon transform the paradigms of healthcare is through the increased use of artificial intelligence (AI) in clinical decision-making. AI aims to mimic the human decision-making process, which according to the dual process theory, there are two types: Type I and Type II.[11] Type I refers to fast, reflexive decision-making processes based on intuition, whereas Type II refers to analytical decision-making. As physicians, we spend much of our time in the Type I, intuitive mode of decision-making, but this mode of decision-making is also where we are most affected by our cognitive biases, which leads to clinical errors. The use of AI in clinical decision-making may allow for the ability to quickly process a huge amount of data using a Type II analytical decision-making process with the speed of a Type I decision. Therefore, a huge amount of data can be rapidly analyzed without the potential for implicit bias, improving patient outcomes. In addition, AI programs may relieve the clerical burden faced by physicians and make sense of the tremendous amount of data that are being inputted into electronic health records to generate clinically relevant information.

As AI continues to gain relevance, physicians will continue to be a part of the decision-making process, although much of the data processing may be done by a computer. Furthermore, the physician's role as an empathic communicator with patients is likely to expand, as social and emotional skills will become more important with increased automation.[12] The physician–patient relationship will remain the core of the medical profession, as the success of providing care is dependent on collaboration, empathy, and shared decision-making. AI may improve the efficiency of healthcare delivery but will not replace the human element of medicine. It may also allow physicians to specialize further by removing or minimizing time spent on routine or administrative tasks, which can take up to 70 percent of a physician's time. We currently spend an inordinate amount of time learning and performing diagnostic skills (algorithmically assisted decision-making) and performing clerical and administrative work. Yet, as technology develops, the medical professional will be able to broaden their focus in patient care and make groundbreaking strides in research, prevention, gerontology, and personalized medicine, enriching the lives of patients.

As medical professionals, we must acknowledge that the paradigms of healthcare have changed throughout history and will continue to change in the future. We must recognize that our roles and responsibilities may change as a result. However, instead of experiencing overwhelming anxiety or discontent due to these changes, we should work to manage our expectations and recall our commitment to lifelong learning. Understand that change is likely to ultimately be good; for example, AI and telehealth will likely allow us to deliver better care and ensure greater health for society. Furthermore, be empowered by the fact that no change will take away what makes medicine so special—the human element of connecting with and caring for patients.

Chapter Quick Summary

- Our role as physicians is constantly changing.
- The COVID-19 pandemic is likely to be an important turning point for the medical profession.
- The long-term mental trauma and burden of chronic disease associated with COVID-19 will necessitate changes within the profession.
- One current issue in healthcare is physicians experiencing moral distress due to conflicts between their duty as employees and their ultimate duty to patients.
- Imminent changes in the profession are coming due to incorporation of technology.
- In particular, artificial intelligence and telehealth are likely to have a major impact on our changing roles as physicians.

Resources

AMA STEPSForward. "Telemedicine" [Course]. *AMA EdHub.* October 7, 2015. https://edhub.ama-assn.org/steps-forward/module/2702689

Evans, J.E. "The Changing Ethics of Health Care." *Caring for the Ages.* July 2016. https://www.caringfortheages.com/article/S1526-4114(16)30143-3/pdf

Phillips. "How Will COVID-19 Change the Working Lives of Doctors and Nurses?" April 14, 2020. https://www.philips.com/a-w/about/news/archive/blogs/innovation-matters/2020/20200414-how-will-covid-19-change-the-working-lives-of-doctors-and-nurses.html

References

1. Densen, P. "Challenges and Opportunities Facing Medical Education." *Trans Am Clin Climatol Assoc* 122 (2011): 48–58.
2. Kohli, P., and S.S. Virani. "Surfing the Waves of the COVID-19 Pandemic as a Cardiovascular Clinician." *Circulation* 142, no. 2 (2020): 98–100. https://doi.org/10.1161/CIRCULATIONAHA.120.047901

3. Lai, J., S. Ma, Y. Wang, Z. Cai, J. Hu, N. Wei, J. Wu, H. Du, T. Chen, R. Li, H. Tan, L. Kang, L. Yao, M. Huang, H. Wang, G. Wang, Z. Liu, and S. Hu. "Factors Associated with Mental Health Outcomes among Health Care Workers Exposed to Coronavirus Disease 2019." *JAMA Network Open* 3, no. 3 (2020): e203976–e203976. https://doi.org/10.1001/jamanetworkopen.2020.3976

4. Emami, A., F. Javanmardi, N. Pirbonyeh, and A. Akbari. "Prevalence of Underlying Diseases in Hospitalized Patients with COVID-19: A Systematic Review and Meta-Analysis." *Arch Acad Emerg Med* 8, no. 1 (2020): e35.

5. Skinner, D.E., C.P. Saylors, E.L. Boone, K.J. Rye, K.S. Berry, and R.L. Kennedy. "Becoming Lifelong Learners: A Study in Self-Regulated Learning." *J All Health* 44, no. 3 (2015): 177–182.

6. Gibler, K., O. Kattan, R. Malani, and L. Medford-Davis. "Physician Employment: The Path Forward in the COVID-19 Era." *McKinsey & Company*. July 17, 2020. https://www.mckinsey.com/industries/healthcare-systems-and-services/our-insights/physician-employment-the-path-forward-in-the-covid-19-era

7. Cherny, N.I., B. Werman, and M. Kearney. "Burnout, Compassion Fatigue, and Moral Distress in Palliative Care." In *Oxford Textbook of Palliative Medicine.* 5th ed. Edited by N.I. Cherny, M. Fallon, S. Kaasa, R.K. Portenoy, and D.C. Currow. New York: Oxford University Press, 2015. https://doi.org/10.1093/med/9780199656097.003.0416

8. Shanafelt, T.D., L.N. Dyrbye, C. Sinsky, O. Hasan, D. Satele, J. Sloan, and C.P. West. "Relationship Between Clerical Burden and Characteristics of the Electronic Environment With Physician Burnout and Professional Satisfaction." *Mayo Clin Proc* 91, no. 7 (2016): 836–848. https://doi.org/10.1016/j.mayocp.2016.05.007

9. Deleting Online Predators Act of 2006. H.R.5319, 109th Congress (2005–2006). https://www.congress.gov/bill/109th-congress/house-bill/5319

10. Paul, D.L. "Collaborative Activities in Virtual Settings: A Knowledge Management Perspective of Telemedicine." *J Manage Infor Sys* 22, no. 4 (2006): 143–176.

11. Shea, N., and C.D. Frith. "Dual-Process Theories and Consciousness: The Case for 'Type Zero' Cognition." *Neurosci Conscious* 2016, no. 1 (2016): niw005. https://doi.org/10.1093/nc/niw005

12. Bughin, J., E. Hazan, S. Lund, P. Dahlstrom, A. Wiesinger, and A. Subramaniam. "Skill Shift: Automation and the Future of the Workforce." *McKinsey Global Institute.* May 2018. https://www.mckinsey.com/~/media/mckinsey/industries/public%20and%20social%20sector/our%20insights/skill%20shift%20automation%20and%20the%20future%20of%20the%20workforce/mgi-skill-shift-automation-and-future-of-the-workforce-may-2018.pdf

Index

difficult patients, communication with, 100–1
digital professionalism
  digital communication with patients, 80–81, 101–2
  electronic health records, 85–86
  general discussion, 76–78
  overview, 69
  physician presence on social media, 81–84
  searching for patients on Internet, 79–80
  telemedicine, 84–85
digital resources for stress management, 190
Direct PLUS Loan, 244t
Direct Stafford Loan, 244t
disruptive innovation, 50–51
distraction category of coping, 184t
distress, 181–82
divided attention, 262
doctor–nurse–pharmacist team, 144
Does level, Miller's pyramid, 9–11, 11f
drug abuse. *See* substance use disorders
dual process theory, 24
duty to report, 203–4
Dweck, C., 182
dysthymia, 199

economic issues related to AI, 55–58, 56b
educational debt, managing, 243–47, 244t, 245b
electronic health records (EHRs), 52, 54, 85–86
Ellis, A., 185–86
Emmons, R.A., 36t, 186
emotion-focused coping, 183
emotions, effective communication of, 130–31
emotive empathy, 103, 103t
Empathetics course, 108
empathic concern, 107, 107t
empathic distress, 107, 107t
empathy
  bad news, delivering, 95
  components of, 102–4, 103t
  definition of, 104
  developing, 107–8, 109b
  importance of, 63–64, 108–10
  neuroscience of, 105–7, 106f, 107t
  prosocial behavior and, 37
  tools to measure, 104–5
  as universal value, 131

Empathy Exams, The (Jamison), 102
end-of-life care, cultural praxis in, 128, 129b
engagement, 33
Enhanced National CLAS Standards, 126, 127t
Enlitic, 53
Epicurus, 32–33
Erikson, E.H., 8
errors, apologizing for, 99, 100f
escape category of coping, 184t
ethnicity. *See also* cultural praxis
  health disparities, 121f, 121–24, 123b
  of physician workforce versus general population, 124–25
eudaimonic happiness, 32, 35
eulogy exercise, 33–34, 34b
eustress, 181–82
evidence-based practice, 145b
executive functioning, impact of aging on, 262
exercise, 38, 41, 169
exhaustion, in general adaptation syndrome, 180–81
expectation management, 42
experiential learning, 20–21
Experiential Learning: Experience as the Source of Learning and Development (Kolb), 20–21
expertise use, 146

faith. *See* spirituality
family members, treating, 70–71
feedback,
  giving and receiving, 97–98, 98b
  summative feedback, 98
  formative feedback, 98b, 98
fee-for-service healthcare model, 160–61, 248
fellow feeling, 104
FICA Spiritual Assessment Tool, 230
fiduciary relationship, 2
financial considerations
  compensation, changes in, 247–50
  current issues regarding, 240–43
  educational debt, managing, 243–47
  financial illiteracy, 241
  financial resources for physicians, 253
  gender pay gap, 243
  hospital employment versus private practice, 250